W9-BJF-469

PRAISE FOR STEPHEN HYDE AND

PRESCRIPTION DRUGS FOR HALF PRICE OR LESS

"Steve Hyde emerged in the 1980s as a recognized leader in providing innovative, high-quality, and more affordable healthcare. His efforts challenged the norm, but helped establish a nationwide trend that was both beneficial and sustainable. His persistent quest for new approaches has now turned to prescription drugs. We should all heed his thoughts and actions."
—William W. McGuire, M.D., Chairman and CEO, UnitedHealth Group

"For more than thirty years, Steve Hyde has been one of America's most aggressive innovators working to make health care affordable. His solutions for prescription drugs are both simple and revolutionary and will have as profound an impact on prescription drug costs as his health benefit innovations did during the 1980s and 1990s."
—Steve Wiggins, Founder and Former Chairman and CEO, Oxford Health Plans

"I've learned over the years to never underestimate Steve Hyde. This book is just the latest example of his lasting influence on making health care more affordable, a process that has major *negative* implications for both pharmaceutical manufacturers and pharmacy benefit managers."
—Peter Carman, Former Co-Chairman and Global Chief Investment Officer, Citigroup Asset Management

"Steve Hyde is astute, charming, funny, and helpful. Want to save money on pharmaceuticals? Read *Prescription Drugs for Half Price or Less*."
—Regina E. Herzlinger, Professor, Harvard Business School, and author of *Consumer-Driven Health Care*

PRESCRIPTION DRUGS FOR HALF PRICE OR LESS

Stephen S. S. Hyde

BANTAM BOOKS

PRESCRIPTION DRUGS FOR HALF PRICE OR LESS
A Bantam Book / January 2006

Published by Bantam Dell
A Division of Random House, Inc.
New York, New York

The purpose of this book is to provide educational information to the public concerning prescription drugs that are currently prescribed by physicians. It is not intended to be complete or exhaustive or in any respect a substitute for professional medical care. Only a physician or properly licensed healthcare provider can legally prescribe these drugs, their dosages, and the frequency of their use. This book also provides educational information concerning over-the-counter drugs and their use as possible substitutes for prescription drugs. In no event should a patient stop taking currently prescribed drugs nor should he/she substitute over-the-counter drugs for currently prescribed prescription drugs without first consulting his or her properly licensed physician or healthcare provider.

Book design by Karin Batten

Library of Congress Cataloging-in-Publication Data is on file with the publisher.

ISBN-13: 978-0-553-38390-4
ISBN-10: 0-553-38390-6

Printed in the United States of America
Published simultaneously in Canada

www.bantamdell.com

BVG   10   9   8   7   6   5   4   3   2   1

For Bill McLeod

CONTENTS

APPENDIX

ACKNOWLEDGMENTS

Many good people contributed to the development of this book. Jim Harding, my longtime friend and colleague, renewed my interest in prescription drug costs several years ago when he showed me a contract between a PBM and one of its clients. It had more hedges than an English garden. Sharon Sherman provided the essentially timed encouragement to write the book. She also introduced me to fellow author Rob Simon who guided me through the process of structuring the book and developing the book proposal. In addition, he found Mary Ann Naples, my literary agent. Mary Ann, a delight to work with, expertly guided me through the maze in finding not just a publisher, but the best publisher for this book. I couldn't be more pleased with her expertise, her style, or her results.

Many thanks go to my longtime friends Peter Carman, Don Carty, Regi Herzlinger, Bill McGuire, Charles Murray, and Steve Wiggins for saying such nice things about me to prospective publishers. I have a lot to live up to.

Philip Rappaport, my editor at Bantam, has been an enthusiastic guide, adviser, friend, and supporter throughout. He also provided the perfect buffer between my geekish fondness for computer technology and the more traditional requirements of the paper-based book publishing process. What a guy! Thanks, too, go to all the wonderful folks at Bantam, who have so enthusiastically embraced this book. Special appreciation goes to Madeline Hopkins, my copy editor, for making me appear literate; and to Mrs.

x ● Acknowledgments

McConathy, my high school English teacher, for my not having provided Madeline with an even heavier workload.

Apologies go to my wife Loren and to my children for all the time this book took away from family endeavors. I'm back!

Despite all this help, any errors are entirely my own. I thank you in advance for telling me about them, for letting me know about your own experiences in obtaining affordable medications and health care, and for any suggestions you have for improving the book. You can reach me through my website at www.hyderx.com.

PART I

WHY PRESCRIPTION DRUGS ARE SO EXPENSIVE

CHAPTER 1

Who Is This Book For? Everybody Who Uses Prescription Drugs

WHY THIS BOOK?

There are two kinds of people in this country: those who take prescription drugs and those who will. The purpose of this book is simple: to show you how you can dramatically cut your cost of prescription drugs. Following the strategies in this book, you can usually save 50–90% on your prescription costs. Are you thinking that this is impossible—or that it's some sort of gimmick? It's not either. The fact is that most people don't know the simple techniques that can easily deliver huge savings on their prescription drugs.

Here's just one example. Lipitor, which is used to treat high cholesterol, is the largest-selling drug in the world—$11 billion in sales each year. One of the most frequent dosages is a single 10 mg tablet taken once a day to reduce LDL cholesterol (the bad cholesterol) by 25–30%. At retail, a thirty-day supply costs about $65. Most people get started on Lipitor when their doctors give them a handful of free samples and a refillable pre-

4 ● Prescription Drugs for Half-Price or Less

scription for twelve thirty-day supplies. Most of these patients go to their local drugstores to get them filled. If they are among the forty-five-million-plus Americans who don't have prescription drug insurance, they have to pay the full $65 every thirty days. Very few of these consumers realize that they have many lower cost options that work just as well. For example:

A Generic Drug. Approximately two-thirds of the consumers taking 10 mg Lipitor can just as safely and effectively lower their LDL cholesterol by taking a similar drug called lovastatin that costs about $43 at retail.[1] **Savings:$22/month over Lipitor (34% savings)**

Lower Cost Drugstore. By shopping around by phone or on the Internet with several different pharmacies, this same generic lovastatin can be purchased for as little as $23 (Costco mail order, no membership required). Also, your local pharmacy may be willing to match such prices in order to keep you as a customer. **Savings: $43/month over Lipitor (66% savings)**

Tablet Splitting. Some patients may find that lovastatin doesn't work as well as Lipitor. For them, their doctors can write prescriptions for a half tablet daily of 20 mg Lipitor, and receive exactly the same medication in the same dose for about $47. **Savings: $28/month over the 10 mg Lipitor (43% savings)**

Over a period of years, these savings add up to thousands of dollars for just this one drug. And there are hundreds of other drugs for which similar savings are not only possible, but easy for the consumer who knows what to do.

With this book, you can and will save hundreds or thousands of dollars in prescription costs. I'm going to give you detailed, essential, and easily implemented information that will enable you to do this. I've been a healthcare insider, entrepreneur, and consumer advocate for thirty-five years. One of my companies, Peak Health Care, introduced health benefit innovations during the 1970s and 1980s that have since become industry standards in their markets, such as insurance coverage for physician office visits, full hospital coverage with no patient cost, and low-cost prescription drug benefits. Both members and their employers saved hundreds of millions of dollars on their healthcare as a result. More recently, my newest company, Hyde Rx Services Corporation, has brought the cost savings techniques of this book to employers and their employees. The result has been that thousands of members along with their employers are saving huge amounts of money for high quality prescription drug benefits. In *Prescription Drugs at Half Price—or Less*, I tell you the techniques that the drug industry doesn't want you to know about, why drugs cost so much, and how you can beat them at their own game.

WHO IS THIS BOOK FOR?

This book is for anyone—insured or not—who wants to pay less money for his or her drugs. It may be you, or your parent, or a good friend who is tired of paying full retail prices for increasingly expensive prescription medications.

1. **Uninsured.** You may be one of the 43 million people in the United States who have no health

insurance coverage, or one of the millions more, like me, whose insurance doesn't cover prescription drugs. You may be one of the 3.4 million U.S. workers who have lost their employer-provided coverage during the past three years;[2] or one of those who will soon lose such coverage. You may be a retiree whose former employer has cut back on prescription drug benefits or eliminated them altogether. This book can save you thousands of dollars.

2. **Medicare Part D Drug Beneficiaries.** You may be on Medicare, which has just initiated Part D drug coverage beginning in 2006, but which covers only about half of the drug costs for the average beneficiary. You may still be left with large out-of-pocket deductibles, copayments, and holes in coverage. Every chapter in this book can help you save a lot of money on what Medicare doesn't cover. Also, Chapter 13 explains Medicare Part D and how to find the right plan for you from among the many plans offered.

3. **High-Deductible Insurance.** You may have high-deductible health insurance that doesn't kick in until after you've spent hundreds or even thousands of dollars each year. Until the deductible is reached, it's the same as having no insurance at all. I can help you save 50–90% on your drugs.

4. **Insurance with High Copayments.** Even if you are one of the lucky ones who has first-rate coverage through your employer, you are undoubtedly finding your copayments are costing

you more and more every year. In many cases, your copayments can actually exceed the total price of the drugs you'll find by using the techniques detailed in this book. That's right, even insured consumers can save a lot of money with this book.

5. **Health Savings Account.** Finally, you may be one of the more than one million Americans participating in employer-sponsored Health Savings Account (HSA) plans.[3] With an HSA, you receive a high-deductible insurance policy combined with an employer/employee-funded savings account which you can use to help pay for the deductible and other out-of-pocket costs. The idea behind HSAs is that, when you're spending money out of your own savings account, you'll feel like you're spending your own money (which you are), and that you will be a more savvy, price-conscious consumer of healthcare services. It's actually an excellent idea, but it practically forces you to become a much more informed, discerning prescription drug buyer. If you have an HSA, the techniques in this book will help make your savings account grow from year to year, rather than shrinking under the burden of ever-higher drug costs.

Regardless of your health insurance status (or lack thereof), you are almost certainly paying more than you need to for your prescription medications. Worse, the high cost of drugs may be preventing you from buying them at all. This book will help you get the drugs you need at the lowest possible cost.

WHY DO DRUGS COST SO MUCH?

Why are prescription drugs so expensive and becoming more so? The U.S. consumer price inflation rate has been running at less than 2.5% for the past ten years, and yet drug costs have been rising by double-digit rates for just as long. And many new drugs are being priced at hundreds or even thousands of dollars *per treatment*. The problem is that drugs are not priced or sold under the same free-market rules that govern almost everything else you buy, from DVD players to cars to food to clothes to, well, almost everything.

Instead of manufacturers and retailers setting competitive prices to attract the business of price-sensitive customers, we have a system where drug companies can set arbitrarily high prices that are paid by insurance companies who have little power over the doctors who actually decide which drugs are prescribed for patients who don't care about cost because most have insurance. As far as the drug companies are concerned, you aren't even the customer. Your doctor is. Don't believe me? Just ask any drug representative who works for a brand name drug manufacturer. And since doctors don't pay for drugs, they have little reason to either know or care how much they cost. I can't imagine a more lucrative business model for any company than to have customers who could care less about the cost of the products they're ordering.

This system is clearly not working for you, because you *are* a price-sensitive customer. You want and deserve to get the best medication at the lowest price.

This book will tell you how.

CHAPTER 2

Know the System to Beat the System

THE CURRENT DRUG PRICING SYSTEM IS IRRATIONAL

A lot of people, myself included, love Hershey's chocolate bars. They cost about sixty cents each, and people buy them by the boatload. Many can't imagine ever eating any other chocolate bar. So here's my advice to the Hershey company on how they can increase their revenues by almost *a hundred times*—overnight. All they have to do is increase the price of each Hershey bar to $55. That would make them one of the most profitable companies in the history of the planet.

What's that you say? Where ever did I come up with such a cockamamie idea? I got it from an article in the *Wall Street Journal* reporting that the Italian drug company Sigma-Tau had just increased the price of its cancer drug Matulane from 60¢ to $55 per pill.[1] So if a drug company can do it, why can't Hershey? It's obvious, of course, why Hershey can't do it. Nobody would pay $55 for a candy bar, especially when store shelves are laden with competitive products for 1% of the price. So how can Sigma-Tau think it will get away with such an obviously irrational move? The answer goes a long way toward explaining why healthcare costs in general, and prescription drug costs specifically, are so high and getting higher at a record rate.

The current system of high-cost drugs is based on a single, aberrant economic principle. Most consumers neither know nor care about the actual prices of their drugs. That's because their insurance companies have long paid most of their prescription bills, leaving the consuming patients to pay only nominal copayments. Copayments were usually set at fixed dollar amounts, so patients had no need to know or care whether their drugs actually cost $20 or $200. Likewise, doctors, who write the prescriptions, but don't pay for them, have no need to worry about drug prices.

Stuck with most of the bills, including those for Sigma-Tau's Matulane, are the anonymous insurance companies, along with the employers and HMOs that have been able to do little to keep doctors from prescribing expensive drugs at prices that rise far faster than inflation. In the drug manufacturing business, happiness is selling all you can make and never mentioning price.

Patients see drug ads on TV and then go ask their doctors for them. Most doctors not only write the prescription, but give out handfuls of free samples provided by the 90,000 drug representatives who line up to generously stock doctors' sample shelves.[2] These "free" drugs are, quite simply, among the most expensive drugs on the market. Free samples are like a free lunch. There's no such thing.

But, you say, surely the insurance companies and

HMOs should be able to use their massive buying power to make the drug manufacturers set their prices at a more moderate level. Unfortunately, too many insurance companies have been only too happy with the current system.

All they have to do is pass on these costs to their clients—with their own markups—in the form of ever-higher insurance premiums. Even worse, many insurance companies actually receive rebates paid by the drug manufacturers to reward them for promoting more expensive drugs than their members really need. As long as they all do it, there is no incentive to really control costs.

Employers have never been happy with the rising cost of prescription drugs, but they have always had a secret weapon that allowed them to compensate. They just pay their employees less than they otherwise could have to make up the difference. Employees rarely notice—since it is happening to everyone everywhere, this actually appears normal.

But the story gets worse.

The past two decades have seen the rise of a new kind of prescription drug middleman called the pharmacy benefit manager or PBM. PBMs promise lower drug costs to their employer and insurance company clients. They do this by pooling the combined purchasing power of millions of patients to force the drug retailers and manufacturers to sell drugs to the PBMs at lower prices. The PBMs then pass these lower prices on to their clients—at least in theory.

As it turns out, the drug manufacturers were only too happy to play along with this new PBM development. They could easily accommodate a 15% discount to the PBMs by simply raising drug prices by 20%. The drug companies became even happier when they discovered they could get the PBMs to actually promote their most expensive drugs by paying them rebates instead of providing discounts. Since PBMs didn't have to pass these cash kickbacks through to their clients, this made the PBMs very happy, and most of their clients didn't know enough to ask for their share. And even when some clients learned to ask, they found that the PBMs were unwilling to give them details of their deals with the drugmakers.

PBMs also learned that they can make a lot of money by selling drugs from their own mail order pharmacies and by keeping part of the retail pharmacy discounts they were so successful in negotiating. In fact, PBMs actually lose a lot of money on the fees they charge their clients for claims processing and other administrative services. But despite such loss leader services, the rebates, retail markups, and mail order profits have made the PBM business very profitable indeed.

None of this adds up to an incentive for PBMs to provide their clients and members with the drugs they need at the lowest possible cost. In fact, it is quite the opposite. Instead of becoming the price-busting intermediaries between the client and the vendors, the PBMs have become drug distributors themselves, adding yet another expensive link to the drug distribution chain. Whatever you can say about PBMs, they have not been fiduciaries that try to provide their clients with the drug benefits they need at the lowest possible price.

What about the pharmacies themselves? The PBMs have forced them to provide discounts from their normal prices, and there is little the pharmacies can do about it. Pharmacies have little or no control over what doctors prescribe and patients purchase. For the most part, they are just passive links in the drug distribution chain. But even the smaller profit percentage allowed the pharmacies by PBM-negotiated pricing adds up to a lot of money on the pharmacies' bottom lines, especially when drug prices are going up by 15–19% per year. And the drugstore can always put the pharmacy in the back of the store, so that consumers will also buy flowers, toothbrushes, and motor oil on their way to pick up their prescriptions.

This all adds up to prescription drugs being the most out-of-control cost in healthcare. Drugs represented less than 5% of total healthcare costs in 1980, 10.6% in 2003, and are predicted to balloon to nearly 15% of total costs by 2011.[3] In dollar terms, we spent $12 billion in 1980, $122 billion in 2000, $141 billion in 2001, and $180 billion in 2003.[4,5] It's out of control, and you're bearing more than your fair share of the pain.

Even insured patients are no longer seeing small $5 and $10 copayments for expensive drugs. Instead, they have to pay $25, $50, or more. Many have to pay 100% of drug costs up to a deductible limit, and still others pay a fixed percentage of their drug prices.

The pain is increasingly felt by all drug consumers. The uninsured have been hit with the full brunt of prescription drug costs that have soared beyond any relationship to patients' income or to low levels of inflation in the rest of the economy. Self-pay patients are stuck with paying full price. Some have had to choose between drugs and food. The insured, while better off, are seeing more of the cost burden being transferred to their shoulders as insurers and employers are implementing deductibles, raising copayments, reducing coverage limits, and switching to percent-sharing coinsurance plans. All drug consumers are looking for alternatives to high drug costs.

This book is for these people, for the insured and

the uninsured who want to get the drugs they need at the lowest possible prices.

WHY DOCTORS PRESCRIBE WHAT THEY DO

I mentioned earlier that the drug companies consider the doctor, not the patient, to be the actual customer for their drugs. This reality is based on a simple legal fact: no prescription drug can be purchased by a consumer until some physician (or other similarly licensed health professional) has prescribed it. To understand why you pay so much for the drugs your doctor has prescribed, it helps to know why doctors prescribe what they do. Like many patients, you probably believe that your doctor learns about the drugs he prescribes from reading about scientific drug research in medical journals, or perhaps from discussions with his colleagues and from his own experience prescribing drugs to his patients. This explanation is essentially correct, but far from complete.

What influences a doctor in deciding to prescribe a medication?

Medical literature

Independent medical journals regularly publish the results of trials of medications in the treatment of disease. These articles are rigorously checked by independent expert referees to determine that the author has the qualifications and the experimental rigor necessary for publication in the journal. Increasingly, they are also asking about the researchers' independence from drug company influence. As a result, doctors place justifiable credibility in such articles, whether published in the prestigious *New England Journal of Medicine, Lancet, Journal of the American Medical Association* (JAMA), or one of scores of other journals.

Unfortunately, the sheer volume of new literature is overwhelming to a doctor with a busy practice and limited time for professional reading. Doctors have to prioritize what they read and how much time they spend on an article. The result is that many useful articles receive only cursory attention, if any, leaving the doctor only partially armed with the latest information. This sad state of affairs contributes to a widespread lack of consistency of practice from one doctor to another.

Medical conferences

Many doctors attend medical conferences in an effort to stay current in their fields. Many of these conferences feature trade shows or prominent sponsorships in which drugmakers and other vendors vie for the physician's attention and prescription pad. Doctors consider these conferences and trade shows to be a useful way to stay current, but they have to endure a deluge of drug promotion in the process. Drug companies do this because it works. Doctors respond to advertising and promotion pretty much like the rest of us—especially when it costs them nothing to do so.

Conversations with colleagues

Doctors learn a lot from discussions, often brief, with their colleagues who have superior knowledge about a specific condition or drug. This is particularly true when the colleague is a specialist in a disease that your doctor may not be as experienced with. A hurried conversation in a hospital lounge, at a medical society meeting, or over lunch is a common means for doctors to learn from a more experienced colleague.

Patient preferences

Doctors are more open to your drug preferences than you may have ever imagined. You may be surprised to learn that 69% of all patients who ask their doctor for a specific brand name drug actually get it.[6] This is powerful confirmation that doctors listen to patients and want to keep them happy whenever possible. Unfortunately, this often works against patients who only know to ask for the drugs they've seen advertised on television. These drugs are always expensive. They have to be in order to pay for almost $4.5 billion a year in consumer advertising.[7] In the next chapter, you will learn seven key questions to ask your doctor to make sure you get the best AND lowest cost drugs for your needs.

Drug company promotion

If you think drug companies pay a lot to advertise to you, you may be surprised to learn they spend much more on advertising and promotion to doctors.[8] That way, when you walk into your doctor's office and ask for the Megamycin you saw advertised on TV, your doctor will not just know about it. He'll also be able to give you a handful of "free" samples to get you started.

All together, drug companies spend somewhere between $15 billion and $21 billion a year on advertising and promotion.[9] And it works. Such promotional efforts have become increasingly frenzied over the years as more and more "me-too" drugs have appeared on the market that offer little or no differentiation from similar drugs already being sold—sometimes for a tenth the price. Where once there may have been only a single drug available for a particular condition, there are now often five or more similar drugs with similar effects, each vying for a place of prominence on the doctor's prescription pad. Competition among these products is intense.

In this marketing battle, the drug companies use three primary mechanisms to influence doctors' prescribing habits: direct doctor promotion of brand name drugs, direct consumer promotion of brand name drugs, and drug formulary management. I'll give you a brief rundown on each. You will note the conspicuous absence of price as a competitive tool for brand name drugs.

HOW DRUG MANUFACTURERS SELL THEIR WARES

Direct doctor promotion

The spearhead for drug company promotion is the manufacturer representative, or drug rep. There are 90,000 of these drug company employees roaming the country; their sole job is to meet with doctors and spin as positive a story about their particular drugs as they legally can, so that these doctors will prescribe them by name.[10] They arrive at the doctor's office well armed with free pizza, pens, calendars, knickknacks, gewgaws, tchotchkes, and technical data on their drugs' effectiveness and safety, not to mention thousands of dollars worth of free samples. Next time you visit a doctor, try to count all the items in his exam room containing the name of a brand name drug.

Many doctors value drug rep information, because it represents a faster, easier, and more current way to get information than digging out and reading journal articles. Doctors suffer from an explosion of information in their fields, and their time is precious. Well-informed, honest drug reps can be a useful source of information. It is never far from the rep's mind, however, that her bonus depends on convincing her assigned doctors to increase the number of prescriptions they write for her drugs. This can bias the objectivity of the rep in determining what information to present.

Many other doctors are shunning this plague of drug reps entirely, on the basis that they are counter-productively biased and time-consuming. The Duke University School of Medicine has even adopted a No Free Lunch program with the motto, "Just Say No to Drug Reps." They have announced a "Pen Amnesty" program, in which doctors can turn in their drug advertising writing instruments for officially logoed No Free Lunch pens—no questions asked.

Still, many doctors now get most of their information on drugs from drug reps. Since these salespeople are under intense pressure to produce sales, not all of them stick to the script when they are within the confines of a doctor's office, and sometimes it's the rep's employer who is pushing a tainted script on the rep. Such transgressions can range from simple exaggeration, to suggestions for off-label use (sometimes with the company's endorsement), to outright false claims about a drug's proper uses and effectiveness.[11,12]

It is little known outside the industry that drug-makers and their reps have access to weekly prescriber reports that reveal exactly how many prescriptions each doctor prescribes for the rep's drugs as well as for the competition's.[13] Drugstores sell this information to data aggregators that sell it to the drug companies. The pharmaceutical companies pay dearly for this information, and use it to gauge the effectiveness of their drug reps. Since the drug reps are assigned specific territories consisting of specific doctors, the reps' employers have a powerful tool to motivate and measure each rep's sales performance. If a doctor fails to prescribe enough of a particular drug, the responsible drug rep can find his compensation, and ultimately his career, endangered. Many doctors don't even know that such prescriber reports are available. I don't know of another industry where each producer has access to such perfect, detailed information about its and its competitors' sales information.

A key tool drug reps use to push their drugs is the "gift" of free samples for the doctors to give to their patients. Drug reps practically shovel these pills into doctors' sample closets. A quick tour of a typical doctor's sample supply will reveal a mini-drugstore with many thousands of dollars worth of expensive drugs. Rare is the patient who hasn't been given a handful (or bag full) of medications from her doctor, along with a prescription for more of the same.

Sampling is an effective way to get patients started on a drug to see how it works before starting to pay at the drugstore. In fact, samples are sometimes referred to by drug companies as "starters." Samples have proved to be a powerful influence on what doctors prescribe, since a doctor is much more likely to specify a drug that he can get the patient immediately started on.

Generic drugs, the lowest cost prescription drugs, are rarely provided to doctors as samples. This reduces the likelihood that a doctor will prescribe them.

Drug manufacturers actively promote their products to doctors through advertising in medical journals and through sponsorship of continuing medical education and a plethora of activities at medical conventions.

Interestingly, one piece of information that is almost never included in these promotions is the price of the drug. And doctors rarely ask. After all, doctors don't have to pay for it, and in most cases patients don't ask, but if they did, doctors might learn to find the answer. As discussed above, insurance companies and government programs pay most of the bills. This mentality has allowed the drug manufacturers to price their products with little or no concern for cost-conscious prescribers or consumers. This is why their periodic, breathtaking price increases bear no relationship whatever to the general rate of inflation in the economy.

Direct to patient promotion

In 1997, the FDA loosened restrictions on what drug companies can say in consumer drug advertisements. As a result, direct-to-consumer drug ads have exploded, with ad spending tripling to almost $2.5 billion by 2001 and then to $4.5 billion by 2004.[14]

Are these companies crazy? Everybody knows that doctors decide what to prescribe, not their patients. That's why we have doctors, to evaluate our symptoms, come up with diagnoses, consider all the treatment options, and finally to objectively prescribe the best treatment. Then why would the drug companies spend so much money to get their stories to consumers?

You already know the answer. They do it because it works. The drug industry has learned that patient preferences have a powerful effect on what their doctors prescribe. Last year, the FDA reported that in nearly one-fourth of all doctor visits, patients asked for a specific prescription medication they had learned about from direct to consumer advertising.[15] And as I related above, such requests are honored by doctors more than twice as often as not. Doctors want to keep their patients happy.

There is an alternate explanation, however. Maybe it just means that patients are much more savvy at diagnosing their own ills and coming up with appropriate treatments than we've ever given them credit for. But even if that is true, it also means that these ads unnecessarily drive up the costs of prescription medications, because patients are only seeing ads for the expensive drugs, not the low-cost ones that can work just as well. The much cheaper generic medications get virtually zero advertising support from drug manufacturers. So while a patient may indeed conclude that he needs a medication *like* the one advertised on TV, he remains blissfully unaware that an equally safe and effective medication may be available for one-tenth the price of the advertised brand. Later, I'll show you how to deal with this.

All these billions of dollars of consumer advertising, like the advertising to doctors, are as significant for what they *don't* tell—a drug's price. Have you ever seen a TV or print ad for a brand name drug in which the price was even suggested? Neither have I. The drug manufacturers are aiming these ads at people with insurance plans that require them to pay only a fixed-dollar copayment of $25–50 or so, *no matter how much the drug actually costs*. It's not that these consumers don't care about price; it's just that, to them, the copayment *is* the price. They don't care whether the drug itself costs $35 or $350, because their insurer or employer is paying the difference.

I believe that within the next ten years or so, drug companies are going to be competing like crazy on price for their products without any of the hidden kickbacks, side deals, and manipulations that now serve to drive prices up, not down. Unfortunately, you may not be able to wait that long for reasonably priced drugs. You, as a savvy drug consumer, need to know *now* how to navigate the shoals of the current system in order to get the drugs you need—and *only* the drugs you need—at the lowest possible price.

Insurance formularies

An increasingly powerful determinant of what doctors prescribe is the insurance formulary. Essentially, a formulary is a preferred list of drugs that PBMs and insurance companies would rather see prescribed for their patients. Formularies were originally created as a cost-saving measure to allow patients to pay lower copayments for preferred, lower priced drugs—particularly generics. However, the brand name drug manufacturers quickly figured out they could get their most expensive drugs on these formularies by paying the PBM a substantial rebate or kickback on any such drugs purchased by their members. Rebates, combined with drug manufacturer promotion, now have the egregious effect of driving patients away from drugs that promise huge cost savings for themselves, their insurers, and their employers. Many industry observers, including this one, are of the opinion that rebates have complicated and corrupted what began as a valid approach to patient-centered, prescription drug cost savings.

One of the least savory aspects of rebates is that these under-the-table discounts are not available to people who pay for their own drugs. Fortunately, anyone who makes the effort to become a savvy Rx shopper can often circumvent this problem and actually end up paying less for their drugs than patients who have insurance.

By the way, doctors often *hate* formularies. There are scores, perhaps hundreds, of formularies, each with its own unique list of preferred drugs. There is no practical way for your doctor to know whether a given drug is on any given formulary, unless he can access your formulary electronically or you take a copy with you to your appointment. If you don't, they often unintentionally prescribe non-preferred drugs. Patients are usually ignorant of these technicalities, and don't find out until their pharmacists give them the bad news that the drugs prescribed either aren't covered or require a much higher copayment.

It is not a friendly system, but take heart. I'll walk you through some simple steps to get you where you want to be—with the drugs you need at the lowest possible cost.

Generic Drugs Explained

Any brand name drug manufacturer, during the period when a brand is covered by patent exclusivity, has a legal monopoly on the manufacturer and sale of that drug. That's why it can price the drug many times above its production cost. But once a brand name drug loses its twenty-year patent exclusivity, any drug manufacturer is allowed to manufacture and sell it, provided that it meets the same stringent FDA requirements for equivalence, safety, and effectiveness as the original brand name drug.

As a result, where the original brand was controlled and made by a single company, you are likely to have many different companies making a particular generic drug. For example, where Prozac, the blockbuster brand name depression medication, was made solely by Lilly when it was still under patent, I recently counted no fewer than twenty drug companies now making the generic version of the same drug. When this happens, there is only one effective way that any of these manufacturers can compete—by quoting a lower price to the distributors that sell it to the drugstores that actually dispense the drug. The reason you never see a manufacturer advertising or promoting their generic drug to consumers and doctors is that they have no way of assuring that the resulting prescriptions will be filled with their drug. A patient may ask for, and a doctor may write a prescription for fluoxetine (the generic name for the active ingredient in Prozac), but neither has any way of knowing which manufacturer's version will actually be dispensed by the pharmacist. Thus, there is no benefit to a generic drugmaker to advertise or promote its drug to doctors and patients.

When you combine this promotional vacuum for generics with the billions of dollars spent in promoting the brand name drugs to doctors and patients, you end up with a strong bias in favor of doctors prescribing the brands, and an increasing marginalization of generics that are as effective as the brands. In the end, the brand name drug sells big and the generic doesn't.

In Chapter 7, I'll show you the eight steps by which the brand name companies minimize generic use, and how you can turn this to your advantage.

SO, WHOSE FAULT IS THIS?

By now, you have probably concluded that the drug companies are the demons in this story. Or the PBMs. Or the insurance companies. Or the doctors. Actually, there are no evildoers in this story. Virtually every insurance executive, PBM manager, drug company representative, or doctor I've ever met appeared to be a genuinely good person who felt he was doing something positive for his customers, patients, and society. These people are certainly not like the cynical cigarette company executives who, for decades, hid the evidence that their products are both addictive and deadly. Prescription drug manufacturers have arguably done more to extend and enhance lives than has any development since agriculture. True, they engage in behavior that many see as price gouging, but this can also be explained as the most rational response to the rules of an irrational system.

　Is technology the demon? After all, we are deluged with reports on how unbridled technology is driving healthcare costs through the roof. We see all those estimates that the cost of developing a single new drug runs somewhere between $800 million to $1.7 billion dollars—for ONE drug.[16,17] I have never bought this technology-is-the-problem argument. I challenge you to name one other major industry in this country in which technology hasn't driven costs down, way down. OK, not counting the defense industry. My teenage son has a pocket music player with 7,700 songs on it that has more computing power than existed in the entire world in the early 1950s, and with more computer disk memory than was available anywhere until relatively recently. It cost $400 when he bought it last year. If it were a medical device, you would expect that next year it would cost a lot more. But as a consumer product it assuredly won't. Instead, it will get better and better and become cheaper and cheaper.

So who do we blame for the high cost of prescription drugs? To find the real demon in this story, we have to go back more than a half century to World War II. U.S. companies were suffering from a labor shortage as the war machine sucked up millions of young, productive men to do battle with enemies on multiple international fronts. Government wage and price controls prevented these employers from using higher wages to compete for the remaining workers. Instead, employers prevailed on the IRS to issue a then-obscure ruling that allowed them to provide health benefits to their workers without the workers having to pay income taxes on them. This, combined with the fact that the workers couldn't themselves buy the same amount of health services with pretax dollars, led to the utterly perverse situation we have now of employers deciding what health services we can have, and then presiding over a system where the authority lies with the doctor, the responsibility to pay with the employer (via the insurance company), and the ultimate accountability with the patient. As a result, healthcare is the only major industry in our consumer-driven economy (other than defense) that utterly fails to operate within the incentives of our price-driven, free-market economy.

Given the irrational set of rules by which they are required to operate, the drug companies, like other purveyors of healthcare products and services, are actually behaving quite rationally and logically, except of course when such behavior spills over into fraud and illegality. The problem is that this behavior is also schizophrenic. On the one hand, the drugmakers are responsible for the development and sale of wonderfully life-saving, life-enhancing, life-extending miracles from which we all benefit. On the other, they have increasingly engaged in product development and sales behaviors that have resulted in conflicts of interest, inefficiencies, secret payoffs, virtual bribery, false reporting, phony claims, and outright criminal conduct.[18] Not to mention annual cost increases of 15–19%. Even when legal, what may be rational for the drug companies has become punitive for the rest of us.

MANY DRUG CONSUMERS DON'T REALLY NEED DRUGS

One of the more irrational aspects of the system is that many consumers end up taking prescription drugs they don't need. It is surprisingly common for doctors to prescribe unnecessary drugs. For example, a 1995 U.S. Centers for Disease Control study found that more than 40% of all antibiotics were prescribed inappropriately for viral rather than bacterial infections, even though they don't work against viruses.[19] Up to 80% of ear infections and 69% of uncomplicated sinus infections get better without antibiotics.[20,21]

Then there are the many so-called self-limiting

diseases that, with a modicum of time and a healthy immune system, will resolve themselves quite nicely without prescription medications. Colds and their associated misery, minor wounds, many infections, situational stress, occasional insomnia, muscle strains and sprains, and hangovers are to varying degrees amenable to tincture of time, perhaps with the assistance of over-the-counter symptom relievers, home remedies, and moderated behavior.

Yet doctors seem more than willing to prescribe medications for such conditions. This is particularly true for children. A pediatrician friend once told me that fully 30% of his patient visits didn't really require a doctor. These cases mostly involved worried parents wanting to make sure nothing was seriously wrong with their children, and then expecting a pill to fix whatever the actual problem was or potentially could be.

Why does this happen? More often than not, it is because the patient makes it known that he expects (or demands) something, anything, to make him feel better. Doctors want to make their patients happy. So, they will often prescribe something they figure to be marginally useful but harmless. Adding to this tendency is the fact that the doctor doesn't have to pay for the medication, and if the patient doesn't care about cost, why not? At best, such prescriptions constitute very expensive placebos that produce equally expensive urine, and not much more. Occasionally, they do positive harm.

I'm not saying you shouldn't see your doctor when you're ill. Unless you are confident in your self-diagnostic abilities, you may still want a doctor to tell you whether you have a minor skin infection or a flesh-eating staphylococcus bug that requires massive intervention. And doctors and their associated professionals are still the only people who can order a prescription drug, if that's what you really need. It's always a good idea, though, to keep any hypochondriacal tendencies in check. That can be a very expensive disease.

This brings up the subject of self-diagnosis and treatment with the assistance of television advertising.[22] Widely criticized for creating unnecessary demand for expensive drugs, all those billions in consumer drug advertising have also been credited with causing millions of patients to visit their doctors when they might not have otherwise. Sometimes these visits have led to the diagnosis of serious disease.[23] Much of the time, however, the patient is just seeking help for a problem they already know they have. An FDA doctor survey recently confirmed that almost 90% of patients who asked for a specific brand name drug actually had the condition the drug treats. Patients tend to be much savvier than pundits are willing to credit.

The problem occurs when patients walk into the doctor's office asking for a particular drug, instead of help in finding the best, most cost effective way to treat the condition. There is a huge list of individual maladies that respond quite well to disciplined lifestyle changes—without any drug intervention. These conditions include high cholesterol, various pains, high blood pressure, obesity, prediabetes, allergies, stress-related problems, respiratory ailments, and digestive problems. If you smoke, there is not a pill in the world that will prevent your predictable descent into bodily dysfunction, organ failure, cancer, and the ultimate degradation of the quality (and quantity) of your life. Eating a moderate, balanced diet, engaging in regular exercise, foregoing cigarettes, moderating alcohol consumption, and managing stress are all huge contributors to a healthy, prescription-drug-free lifestyle—and with more money to spend on enjoying that lifestyle.

Preaching the evils of smoking, obesity, and personal irresponsibility is not, however, the purpose of this book. Managing the cost of preventing and dealing with the resulting illness is. If you want to save money on drugs, the most basic way is to lead a reasonably disciplined lifestyle that keeps you from needing them in the first place. You don't usually need a doctor to tell you this. At the same time, most people take their doctor's advice seriously, so she can be a good place to start. Just remember that, if you want advice, you need to ask for advice. Asking for a pill is not asking for advice.

Besides cost, there's one more reason to ask your doctor about alternatives to drugs. For many people, prescription drugs can be dangerous—or at least damned unpleasant from unwanted side effects. So many people died after taking Seldane for allergies, Rezulin for diabetes, and Baycol for cholesterol, that the FDA had to remove them from the market. All of these were heavily promoted, huge-selling drugs with side effects that didn't emerge until well after they were approved for sale. Or take Fen-Phen (actually, don't), a combination of two separately approved drugs that many people took to help them lose weight—only to end up with damaged hearts. All of these conditions—allergy, diabetes, cholesterol, and obesity—are often amenable to prevention or treatment for most people by means other than medication, and those means usually involve a lot less expense, not to mention a more active, productive, and fulfilling life.

PART II

IDENTIFYING THE RIGHT DRUGS FOR YOU

CHAPTER 3

Understanding Your Drug Insurance Benefits

Even if you have prescription drug insurance, you are likely paying more than you need to for your drugs. You have probably seen your costs skyrocket from the increased use of deductibles, multitiered co-payments, coinsurance, benefit limitations, and non-covered drugs. Using the techniques in this book, you should be able to save a lot of money. The key is to know your benefits and, particularly, the limits of those benefits. An entire book could be written on this subject, but I have summarized below some of the key elements you need to know. Once you are familiar with your own benefit coverage, the rest of this book will tell you how to make the most of it.

Deductibles are first-dollar amounts that you are responsible for paying before your benefit coverage begins to pay for your drugs or healthcare services. If you do have such a deductible for your drug coverage, be sure to find out if it is a drug-only deductible or whether it is combined with your general medical benefits deductible. The important thing to remember is that, until you pay the entire deductible amount, YOU DON'T HAVE INSURANCE COVERAGE FOR DRUGS. Thus, regardless of how great your coverage may be AFTER the deductible is paid, you should start behaving as a savvy, cost-conscious drug consumer from the start. Then, regardless of the quality of coverage after you've paid the deductible, you will continue to save on your own continuing out-of-pocket drug expenses. Also, make sure you use a participating network pharmacy approved by your insurer. Otherwise, anything you spend at a nonparticipating pharmacy may be excluded or only partially included in calculating how much of your deductible has been satisfied.

Even if you have not yet satisfied your deductible, it is very important that you use your drug insurance card whenever you buy prescription drugs. There are two reasons for this.

1. **Deductible Accounting.** The easiest way for you to make sure your insurance company knows when you have satisfied your deductible is to make sure your pharmacy always uses your card to run your claims through their computer, even if you are paying the entire amount.

2. **Discounts.** Even before you have satisfied your deductible, your drug card will assure that you pay only the discounted price of your drugs negotiated by your insurance company instead of the drugstore's full retail price. The savings can be significant.

Copayments. Over the past twenty-five years, insurance coverage for drugs has increasingly become a completely separate benefit from regular medical coverage. Accompanying this trend has been the rise of PBM benefit administrators and the use of separate, fixed-dollar copayments that patients have to pay for each prescription. In the old days (1980s), you'd be expected to pay a $3 to $5 copayment for any prescription, regardless of the actual cost of the drug.

However, with the explosion in drug prices in the 1990s, PBMs began to use *tiered* copayments. Two-tier copayments were usually $5 for a generic drug prescription and $10 or so for brand name drugs. Then, as drug manufacturers began to pay big rebates to the PBMs for pushing their particular drugs, PBMs invented three-tier structures, where a patient might pay $5 for a generic drug, $10 for a *preferred* (i.e., rebatable) brand name drug, and $15 for a non-rebatable *non-preferred* brand.

Those of you who are now on copayment plans must be looking at these numbers in amazement, since most three-tier copayments are currently running $10–15 for generics, $20–35 for preferred brands, and $35–75 for non-preferred brands. Also, you may well be in a four-tier plan, with even higher copayments (and/or coinsurance) for so-called specialty drugs, such as expensive injectable and biotech drugs.

Increasingly common is an expanded list of drugs that are not covered at all, for which you will have to pay 100% of the cost.

Whatever copayment structure you may have, the concepts in this book can save you a lot of money now, and even more in the future as drug prices continue their stratospheric climb.

Generic Copayments. For plans with fixed-dollar copayments, generic drugs usually provide for the lowest copayment amount, often $10 or so. Be sure to find out if your generic drug copayment is a flat $10, or whether it will be the actual drug cost if that is less than $10. Some programs actually require you to pay the full $10 even if the actual prescription cost is $5. If this is the case with your plan, be sure to ask the pharmacy how much is the drug's cash cost. If it's less than $10, tell them you don't want to use your drug card, but will pay the lower cash amount instead.

Coinsurance. Often combined with a deductible, coinsurance is an insurance industry term for the percentage that you will be required to pay after any deductible is satisfied. For example, if your drug coverage is shown as something like 80/20, that means your insurance company will pick up 80% of the *allowed* amount for your drugs, and you will be required to pay the remaining 20%. Thus, if your prescription is for a month's supply of Nexium for heartburn, the allowed cost of the drug might be $138. You would be required to pay 20% of that amount, or $27.60. You would thus be very interested to know if there were lower cost alternatives that might work just as well for you. And if you do happen to have coverage with only 20% coinsurance for drugs, count yourself lucky. This means you have just about the best drug benefit in the country, especially if there is a cap on the total amount you have to pay in a given year.

Don't be surprised if your employer switches from a fixed-dollar copayment program to a coinsurance program. They are increasingly doing this in order to provide their employees with an incentive to seek the lowest priced drugs that will meet their needs.

If you are under a coinsurance program, then virtually every technique in this book can help you save money.

Participating Pharmacies. Bear in mind that the amount allowed by your insurer will probably apply only when you obtain your drugs through a contracting network pharmacy, so make sure your favorite pharmacy is in the network and will honor the insurer's negotiated price. If you find yourself buying your drugs from a nonparticipating pharmacy, here are the likely penalties you'll have to suffer:

- **Full payment.** When a nonparticipating pharmacy enters your claim in their computer, it is likely to be rejected by your insurer or PBM. That means you'll have to pay the pharmacy the full retail price of the drug up front.
- **Claim submission.** Your coverage may not include out-of-network pharmacies at all, although most insurers will allow you to recover at least part of your cost. This means you will have to fill out a paper claim and submit it with your receipts to your insurer.
- **The wait.** Because over 99% of all pharmacy claims are submitted and adjudicated online and instantaneously, paper claim processing systems tend to be slow and inefficient. You may have to wait weeks for your reimbursement.
- **Limited reimbursement.** Once you receive your reimbursement, if any, you'll need to be prepared to find that your share of the payment will be much higher than if you had used a network pharmacy. There are two possible reasons

for this. First, your insurer's share may be the same *dollar amount* for your drug that it would have paid at a network pharmacy. Remember, you paid full retail for your drug and not the discounted amount available through a network pharmacy, so your share of the payment may well be twice as much or more than if you had used a network pharmacy—especially if you bought a highly marked up generic drug. For example, let's say you filled a prescription for a generic albuterol inhaler for your asthma at a nonparticipating pharmacy at their cash price of $24. If you had purchased it at a participating pharmacy, the allowed cost might have been only $6. Thus, your PBM would require you to pay not only your regular copayment, in this case $6, but also the excess $18 you paid over the allowable amount. In other words, you could end up paying four times as much for a covered drug by going to a nonparticipating pharmacy. Second, for nonnetwork pharmacies, many insurers cover an even lower percentage of the allowed amount for a nonnetwork pharmacy. Thus, if your normal coverage is 80% of the allowed drug cost, it may be only 60–70% of the allowed amount when purchased through a nonnetwork pharmacy. Any way you cut it, wandering into a nonparticipating pharmacy can cost you big time.

Formularies. Also called a preferred drug list, a formulary is a list of drugs that insurers and pharmacy benefit managers (PBMs) and insurance companies would rather see prescribed for their patients. The most frequently encountered formularies are so-called three-tier formularies in which drugs are listed in groups or tiers in order of preference and copayment. Tier 1 usually lists generic drugs, which are usually the lowest cost medications and which require the lowest member copayment amount, perhaps $10 per prescription. Tier 2 drugs are usually preferred brand name drugs that may require a $25 copayment. Tier 3 drugs are nonpreferred drugs with typical copayments of $35 to $75.

Mail Order Drug Benefits. Most drug benefit plans provide an incentive for members who regularly take medications for chronic conditions to buy them from a mail service pharmacy. Such incentives usually allow you to obtain a three-month supply for the equivalent of only twice as much as a retail copayment for a one-month supply. Furthermore, you will not be allowed to get more than a one-month supply at a time at retail. Such plans thus allow you to save up to one-third on copayments for such drugs, and to enjoy the convenience of having a ninety-day supply delivered to your mailbox. Increasingly, though, we are seeing requirements for two and a half times the monthly copayment, reducing the savings to one-sixth of the normal retail copayments. If you're buying a lot of brand name drugs, this could still be a worthwhile savings.

Health Savings Accounts (HSAs). The health savings account is a relatively new form of insurance or insurance-like coverage that many in health care are calling the *new* new thing. Such benefit plans go by a variety of names including Health Savings Accounts (HSAs), Health Reimbursement Arrangements (HRAs), or Medical Savings Accounts (MSAs). Each of these has a different twist on the theme, but incorporate similar features. Here is how these things essentially work.

First, you start with a high-deductible health insurance plan, usually provided by your employer. Rather than the $100 to $500 deductible you may be familiar with, these plans may call for a $3,000 to $5,000 (or higher) deductible, after which the insurance kicks in with a 20–30% coinsurance requirement. Virtually all such plans have a maximum out-of-pocket limit, so that once you have spent the specified amount that year, the insurer then picks up 100% of any allowable medical costs until the end of that calendar year. After that, everything (i.e., deductibles and out-of-pocket maximums) is reset to zero and you start all over again.

The lure of such insurance policies is that they are relatively cheap compared with the far richer plans most insured employees are accustomed to. That makes sense, since these high deductible plans put a much bigger financial burden on the member, so that the insurer's potential liability for paying is much less.

Such high deductible plans, by themselves, would not be particularly attractive to most employees. Also, many employers, particularly the large ones, put a premium on providing a rich, or at least competitive, health benefit plan so that they can attract and keep good workers. Barebones high deductible coverage by itself could make it more difficult for employers to hire top-notch talent.

What distinguishes an HSA or the like from a normal high deductible health plan is the addition of a savings account that can be used to cover a member's deductible and coinsurance costs. It may help to think of the savings account as the medical equivalent of a retirement plan like an IRA or 401(k). Under each, you and your employer can contribute pretax money into a tax-preferred savings account. Unlike the retirement plans, however, the medical savings account allows you to immediately spend up to the current balance of your account for a wide variety of medical expenses not covered by your insurance or health benefit plan. Thus, any deductibles, copayments, coinsurance, or over-the-counter drug costs that are not paid by your insurance can be paid from your savings account.

Let's say that your employer sponsors an HSA plan with a $3,000 annual deductible and that you have elected to participate. Further assume that your employer has agreed to contribute $1000 per year into your savings account. Depending on the actual type of plan, you may additionally be allowed, even encouraged, to contribute your own pretax dollars into the account as well. Let's also say you decide to put in $500 per year, so that the total annual contribution equals $1,500.

Here's how it works. On January 1 of the first year, you wake up with a pain in your back (and likely your head) from overindulging in tabletop dancing the night before. The next day you call your doctor to arrange an appointment. His receptionist would be happy to fit you in to the doctor's schedule sometime in March, or you can see a nurse practitioner that same afternoon. You elect the latter option and are quite happy to find a very competent, caring professional who prescribes tincture of time and prescription-strength ibuprofen that you find is both cheap and effective. The entire bill for your visit is $85 and the prescription ibuprofen costs $5. Because you have $1,500 in your HSA, you are happy to learn that your entire $90 cost is reimbursed by your HSA, leaving $1,410 in the account.

Let's now assume that you enjoy a healthy year and spend nothing else for medical expenses through December 31. You now have a savings account balance of $1,410 (plus any interest or investment income), which is then augmented by an additional $1,500 in contributions by you and your employer in the second year. Since any unused balance in your HSA rolls over from year to year, you find that you now have $2,910 in your account, which is almost equal to the entire amount of your deductible. Thus, if you were to suddenly suffer a catastrophic medical expense—a $100,000 heart surgery, for example—your HSA would pay almost all of your $3000 deductible, and your insurance would pay all of the rest with the exception of any required coinsurance.

The key feature of HSA-like programs is that anything in your savings account at the end of the year rolls over from year to year. Such a residual balance can be invested and earn income without being taxed, as long as it stays in the account or is used for allowed medical expenses. Over a period of years, you have the potential to build it up so that it can cover you completely for any high-cost medical event.

If you happen to have a chronic condition, such as diabetes or high blood pressure, you may find yourself spending the entire amount of your account each year, plus any remaining deductible. Thus if in the above example, you have to spend $2,500 per year on drugs and medical care, then anything in excess of your and your employer's $1,500 annual contribution—i.e., $1,000—will come out of your pocket—until $3,000 has been spent and the insurance kicks in. You obviously have a strong incentive to get your annual expenditures down to $1,500 or less, preferably through savvy shopping for drugs and health services and by living a healthier lifestyle. You might be able to cut costs by cutting your care, but that's almost assuredly a short-term solution that will bite you in your nether regions in the longer run. John Maynard Keynes once said, "In the long run, we're all dead." Presumably, you would like for your own run to be as long as possible.

Regardless of your condition, the idea of the HSA is to give you the incentive to be a cost-conscious consumer of all medical care, and not just prescription drugs. However, since many patients pay more for prescription drugs than for any other medical expense, this book should be at the top of their reading list.

Flexible Spending Accounts. Flexible Spending Accounts (FSAs), also called Part 125 plans or cafeteria plans, allow employees to annually contribute a pretax sum to a designated account to be used to pay for a defined range of benefits, such as over-the-counter drugs or prescription drug copayments that are not otherwise covered by the normal health benefits. At the beginning of each year, the employee specifies how much the employer should withhold from each paycheck to fund his FSA. During the year, the employee can receive reimbursement from this account for most medical expenses not covered by the employer's insurance. There are two big differences between an FSA and the HSAs described above: First, only the employee contributes to the FSA, although with pretax payroll deductions. Second, an FSA is a use-it-or-lose it proposition; any funds remaining at the end of the year are forfeited to your employer and you start the new year with a zero balance. Even with these limitations, FSAs can be an effective way to defray the costs of healthcare and other expenses that you know you will have, as the tax savings can be significant.

Maximum Lifetime Benefit Amounts. Many health insurance plans, including both group and individual policies, have maximum lifetime benefits, such as $1,000,000 or $3,000,000. If you ever hit this limit, your insurance will no longer cover you at all. Generally, the only way to obtain coverage after that is to get a new job (and a new insurance plan), unless you are eligible for Medicare (for seniors and the disabled) or Medicaid (for the poor). Fortunately, lifetime limits are high enough that few people ever experience them.

Maximum Out-of-Pocket Amounts. Most insurance plans, particularly those with large deductibles and coinsurance requirements, provide that you will be liable only for a maximum amount of out-of-pocket payments. After you reach this limit, the insurance usually covers you at 100% of all allowable medical charges.

Know your health insurance benefits. And then use the principles in this book to get the most out of your prescription drug benefits for the least amount of your money.

CHAPTER 4

Consult Your Biggest Allies: 7 Questions to Ask Your Doctor and Pharmacist

Let me tell you a story that is typical of many patients. Before becoming a noninsured member of Hyde Rx, Erin Lee (not her real name), went to her doctor complaining of periodic heartburn, especially after a large meal. After a series of questions and tests, Erin's doctor diagnosed gastroesophageal reflux, a condition involving a flow of acid from the stomach up into the esophagus (your swallowing or food tube). Like tens of thousands of other doctors, Erin's physician gave her a handful of free samples of a drug called Nexium, the "new purple pill" that has been advertised heavily on television and in print. Along with the samples, he gave her a refillable prescription for the drug, which she would need to take for at least several months. Happy to receive something for free, Ms. Lee left the doctor's office only to find at the pharmacy that the prescription itself was going to cost her $138 a month!

This and similar rude shocks hit thousands of patients every day. It starts when they feel hesitant or even intimidated about asking their doctors how much a drug will cost. Most take the prescription, get the bad news at the pharmacy, and either fork over their scarce cash or just walk away without their drugs. They are utterly unaware that they could have spent a lot less money by asking their doctors a few simple questions.

In Ms. Lee's case, she was able to become a member of Hyde Rx, where she learned that most people who take Nexium can do just as well with another drug, Prilosec OTC, which is available over the counter for $15–$20 a month.[1] But how can a drug you buy off a drugstore or grocery shelf be as effective as a prescription drug costing more than six times as much? It's simple, really. Prilosec, like Nexium, used to be available only by prescription and cost about $130 per month. But when Prilosec lost its twenty-year patent protection, its manufacturer decided to begin selling it—in *full prescription strength*—over the counter in order to continue with a profitable, well-known brand name. Nexium, which is actually made by the same company (AstraZeneca), is in reality a modified version of Prilosec—but modified enough for it to receive a new twenty-year patent and the exclusive right to manufacture it. Nexium's clinical testing revealed that Nexium has little if any benefit over its now-cheap predecessor for most patients. And Erin Lee is now saving a lot of money, while getting effective treatment for her acid reflux.

Now Erin doesn't have any drug insurance at all, but even people who do may find themselves paying copayments of $35–50 for a drug like Nexium, despite the fact they could also be buying Prilosec OTC for much less.

In this chapter, I'm going to give you powerful information on how you can work with your doctor to get the drug you need, but at the lowest possible cost. In many cases, that drug will not be the one that's at the top of your doctor's mind, because of all the heavy promotion I discussed earlier. But do not think of your doctor as your adversary in this process. In fact, it is vitally important for you to realize that your doctor is your greatest potential ally in getting the drugs you need at the lowest possible prices. This is true no matter how much insurance you may or may not have. Doctors are increasingly aware of how the drug manufacturers try to manipulate them into prescribing unnecessarily expensive drugs for their patients. You just need to help nudge them in the right direction, and it is *so* easy.

HOW TO TALK TO YOUR DOCTOR

Let your doctor know you don't want to spend any more on drugs than is absolutely necessary. Tell her you don't care whether she prescribes a drug you saw advertised on TV, as long as you get what you need at the lowest possible cost. Chances are your doctor has many patients who tell her this, so she is likely to be surprisingly helpful in saving you money. I probably go to as many different doctors as most people my age, and I have always found them to be willing to go an extra step to help me save money—but only when I ask for their help.

But whether your doctor is knowledgeable or clueless about actual drug costs, there are seven questions you should ask her every time she's about to prescribe drugs. Ask these questions, and you'll most likely walk out of her office with the lowest cost drug bill.

Remember that, in most cases, your doctor can choose from a surprising number of similar medications (or recommend no medication at all) to treat your problem. Prices for alternative meds can vary by a factor of 10 or more. Take the initiative and make sure she knows that cost is an issue for you. Otherwise, the most likely outcome is that she will assume you don't care about cost and give you a few of those incredibly expensive "free" samples and a prescription for more of the same stuff for you to buy later. By the time your pharmacist hits you with the bad news, you will have lost a valuable opportunity to have your doctor work with you to find the most cost-effective treatment plan.

Here are the 7 Questions to ask your doctor. They are explained more fully below and in subsequent chapters.

Doctor, can I save money with:

1. Alternatives to drugs?
2. OTC drugs instead of Rx?
3. Generic drugs?
4. Lower priced brand name drugs?
5. Tablet-splitting doses?
6. Hundred-day mail order Rx?
7. Extra free samples?

Who can actually remember seven questions? Almost nobody, so make a copy of Appendix A at the end of this book. It lists not only the 7 Questions, but also provides a worksheet for you to list all your current medications to take with you on your next doctor visit.

He's probably a reasonably fast reader and might even appreciate the time you've saved him by clueing him in early on your concerns. Showing your doctor a list of your drugs is also a good reminder for him to review all of your current medications, especially if some of your prescriptions are from other doctors. Later in this chapter, I'll provide you with more information on each of these questions, and I'll give you the full background and detail in later chapters.

Will My Doctor Be Upset by All These Questions?

Until I became active in making health care more affordable, I felt the same way about my doctor as most Americans did for much of the past century: that he was on a different plane of existence from me, with godlike knowledge and virtual power over life and death. In many ways, doctors have long been viewed by their patients as being almost like priests. After all, they wear distinctive garments and paraphernalia (e.g., a stethoscope), use a language most of us can't understand, and engage in seemingly ritualistic practices to invoke almost miraculous powers of healing. Many of us just listen to her pronouncements and try to heed her words of infinite wisdom as best we can. In earlier times I would never have thought of questioning anything my doctor said. Today, many patients still accept doctor's diagnoses, decisions, and prescriptions without question or discussion. Some are afraid of offending their doctors, or they just don't want to take up the doctors' precious time.

But many other patients have begun to take more personal responsibility for their own health and treatment, and they want to be active participants in the process. Most doctors are not just open to this more collaborative approach; they welcome it. They get more professional satisfaction from their informed, involved patients. These are the ones most likely to follow her recommendations. They are the patients who not only understand the "what" of the treatment instructions, but the "why," as well. Also, it is really helpful for a doctor to know what a patient is actually willing to do and what he is willing is to pay for. The only way to find that out is for the patient to tell her. So tell her.

A recent survey of doctors revealed that the vast majority (93%) know that drug costs can be a financial burden for many of their patients.[3] The other 7% apparently reside on Mars. Three-quarters of them responded that they believe they have an obligation to initiate conversations on drug costs. Many don't, however, put their beliefs into practice. Common reasons for not doing so turn out to be concerns about patient discomfort, a lack of being able to offer a solution, and the doctors' own discomfort in raising the issue. Doctors don't want to offend their patients by somehow suggesting that they can't afford treatment.

But if the patient raises the issue, this survey makes it clear that doctors are more than willing to help, especially if the patient is asking questions that effectively guide the doctor to good solutions. That's what the 7 Questions provide.

How to Start the Conversation

This new doctor attitude makes it much easier for you to do *the single most important thing* you can do to save money on drugs: tell your doctor you are truly concerned about how much your drugs cost, and that you would appreciate any help he can give you in making sure you get the drugs you need at the lowest possible cost.

You can say something like this, "Doctor, I don't have any (or very much) health insurance, and I'm concerned about how much my drugs are going to cost. I can't afford really expensive medications. Would you please look at this short list of questions to see if you can *help me* save money?" As you ask, hand him the list of 7 Questions from Appendix A. This simple request for help can utterly change your doctor's focus when it comes to prescribing your medications. It can turn him from a virtual—if unintentional—brand name drug salesman into your strongest ally in the fight to secure effective, low cost drugs.

Of course there is always the patient who goes too far, walking into the doctor's office with stacks of Internet printouts and a preconceived diagnosis and treatment conclusion (usually wrong) that he expects the doctor to confirm. This wastes a lot of time and can understandably turn off the doctor.

The best approach is to ask smart, informed questions. If you don't understand something the doctor said, ask him to clarify. If you saw something on the Internet, ask about it, but don't ask him to read the article. If you suspect that your problem may be different from what the doctor has diagnosed, ask specifically about your suspicion. If he says it's just a mole, but you're afraid you have cancer, ask about cancer. In all likelihood, his explanation will relieve your fears while clarifying his diagnosis and recommendations for treatment. Sometimes your question may lead to your disclosure of additional symptoms you didn't think to mention before.

The most important thing to realize is that it's all right to ask questions and to expect your doctor to answer them fully, clearly, and patiently. In thirty-plus years, I've seen a long list of doctors for myself and for my family and friends. Only once in all that time did a doctor literally start backing toward the door when I started asking questions about her diagnosis. We never went back to that doctor. All the rest made sure they addressed our issues, concerns, and questions in a receptive, professional manner. Expect that. And if you don't get it, don't change your approach. Change doctors.

There is another potential benefit to letting your doctor know you are price-sensitive. Instead of charging you for the full price of your patient visit, the doctor may down-code it to a lower fee. Give him a hint and ask what kind of visit he will charge you for. You may save even more.

It is far worse for you to say nothing, and then watch while he writes a prescription or leaves the exam room only to return with a bag of samples and a written prescription for more of the same expensive drugs. Even then, it's not too late to do something about it. You can simply say something like, "I've heard that samples are always expensive when I replace them. Is there a lower cost alternative that could work for me?" Then hand him the 7 Questions.

Hyde Rx's members have done this by the thousands, and I very rarely hear of any doctors resisting this approach, much less taking offense. However, it occasionally happens that a doctor shows some resistance, particularly when she's woefully behind schedule during a really busy Monday with a bunch of impatient patients stacked up in the waiting room. That's why it is important to tell her your concerns and ask the 7 Questions *before* she starts writing your prescription or leaves the exam room. It saves time for you both.

But let's say that you've done all of this in a properly respectful manner, and you still get resistance from your doctor. He may say something like, "This is the best drug for your condition, and you don't want to take any chances, *do you*?" How do you handle that? I would say something like, "So you're saying that you can't use *any* of these methods to help me save money?"

If he still says no, there are two possibilities. The first is that his prescription really is the best for you. If this is the case, your doctor should be able to quickly explain why. Your job is not to second-guess your doctor's expertise; just to make sure he has considered the options and that you understand what you need to do. A second possibility is that he doesn't have the time or doesn't want to take the time to do some research in his Physician's Desk Reference (PDR) that every doctor keeps on his desk or in a handheld computer. If he doesn't try to explain why his prescription is the best, lowest cost approach, or if you're not satisfied with his explanation, there is no point in arguing. Just take the prescriptions and leave. But give some serious thought to finding a new doctor who is more open to your needs.

I've probably spent more words telling you what could go wrong than explaining what is most likely to happen—here's what I have experienced, with variation, every time I've used this approach over the years:

Steve: "Doctor, before you write any prescriptions, I want you to know that I have to pay the entire cost of my drugs, and would appreciate any help you can give me in keeping costs down. Can you look at these *(as I hand him the 7 Questions)* and see if you can help me save money?"

Doctor *(Glancing at my medical record)*: "But I thought you had insurance."

Steve: "I do, but it doesn't cover drugs. (or, "I do, but I still have to pay a big part of my drug costs")

Doctor: "Oh. Well, sure *(and then takes another look at the list)*. Well, we could do this . . . and this."

And so it should go for you virtually every time.

IF YOU HAVE INSURANCE

If you have insurance, find out if it includes a drug formulary or preferred drug list. Chances are that you are on some sort of tiered copayment system, where you pay less for generic and preferred brand name drugs than for non-preferred brand name drugs. Get a copy of this list from your employer's benefits administrator or insurance company. Visit your health benefits administrator at work, or call your insurance company and say, "I would like to get a copy of the drug formulary or preferred drug list for my prescription drug benefit plan." To speed up the process, ask if the formulary is available online at a website, and if it is, find it and print two copies. Keep one copy and give the other one to your spouse. (See sample on the next page.)

Sample Drug Formulary

Bob's HMO and Storm Door Company*

ALLERGY, COUGH, & COLD

Tier 1-Generics	Tier 2-Preferred Brands	Tier 3-Non-Preferred
COPAY $10	COPAY $30	COPAY $50
cyproheptadine	Beconase AQ	Allegra
chlorpheniramine	Zyrtec	Allegra-D
dexchlorpheniramine		Astelin
diphenhydramine		Flonase
guaifenesin/codeine		Nasacort AQ
hydroxyzine		Nasonex
promethazine		Rhinocort AQ

ANTI-SPASTICITY & MUSCLE RELAXANTS

Tier 1 COPAY	Tier 2 COPAY	Tier 3 COPAY
baclofen		Dantrium
carisoprodol		Zanaflex
cyclobenzaprine		

Sample Drug Formulary (cont'd)		
Bob's HMO and Storm Door Company*		
Tier 1-Generics	**Tier 2-Preferred Brands**	**Tier 3-Non-Preferred**
COPAY $10	COPAY $30	COPAY $50
ASTHMA & OBSTRUCTIVE PULMONARY DISEASE		
Tier 1 COPAY	**Tier 2 COPAY**	**Tier 3 COPAY**
albuterol	Advair Diskus	Accolate
ipratropium	Azmacort	Alupent
isoproterenol	Combivent	Flovent
metaproterenol	Foradil	Pulmicort
terbutaline	Proventil HFA	Serevent
theophylline	Qvar	Singulair
	Theo-24	
	Uniphyl	

*Not a real insurance company

Take the formulary list with you whenever you or any family member goes to the doctor. This will allow the doctor to take into account your insurance coverage when prescribing drugs, so that you'll pay the lowest possible copayment. Most doctors will appreciate your doing this, since it prevents them from later getting interrupting calls from the pharmacist asking for a change of prescription because he prescribed a non-covered drug. Always remember, for most common health conditions, he has a wide range of prescribing alternatives. If he can see a list of those drugs that mean the least financial hardship for you, he will be glad to take that into account in prescribing your drugs. Despite all you may have heard or read, doctors are still focused on meeting the needs of their patients first and foremost—and that includes helping you find the right drugs at the lowest cost.

If you forget to take the formulary to the doctor's office or get a prescription you're not sure about, here's what you can do. Before leaving the doctor's office, call the customer service number on your drug ID card (it may be combined with your insurance card) and ask if the prescribed drug is on the preferred drug list. If it's not, find out what comparable drugs are. Then go back to your doctor's nurse (and often you can do all this by phone), explain your problem, and ask if the doctor can change your prescription to a lower cost, preferred drug. Most of the time you will find the doctor willing to do this, but don't be surprised if you hear some grumbling about those damned insurance companies.

THE 7 QUESTIONS EXPLAINED

Here are the critical 7 Questions along with a brief explanation of each, but you'll find much more on all of these in later chapters. I've put them in the order you should ask them, so please take note—this is powerful information. Your prescription costs are going to change for the better!

Question #1: Do I really need any drug at all?
Potential Savings: 100%

Most doctors will love your for asking this question. They are increasingly concerned about patients who demand antibiotics for a cold or flu (useless against such viral diseases), or expect the doctor to just fix whatever they've got with a pill. The fact is that many ailments will heal themselves. This is particularly true for children. Other conditions may be satisfactorily resolved with lifestyle changes. Smoking cessation, exercise, and eating responsibly are the Big Three in this category. Alas, there is no magic pill to replace these.

Nonetheless, many doctors, being eminently human, follow the line of least resistance and prescribe something harmless to placate the patient. At best, these are VERY expensive placebos. At worst, they can cause positive harm from allergic reactions, promotion of antibiotic-resistant disease strains, harmful side effects, and just sheer toxicity. Ask this question and let your doctor know you're not one of those patients.

Question #2: Are there any over-the-counter (OTC) medications that will work?
Potential Savings: 90%

Over the past decade, many very powerful, very safe, and very effective medications have crossed over from prescription to over-the-counter (OTC) status. Two of the most recent and powerful examples are Claritin and its generic sibling loratadine for allergies, and Prilosec for heartburn/acid reflux. Both drugs are not only OTC but also in full prescription strength. As OTC drugs, their prices are a fraction of what they commanded as prescription drugs, and are usually considerably less than even the copayments that insured patients would otherwise have to pay. For example, loratadine (generic Claritin) now costs about $3 for a month's supply in warehouse stores and over the Internet, while prescription Clarinex, a similar drug, costs about $79 for a month's supply. An insured patient might pay a copayment of $25 for a month's supply of Clarinex, and an uninsured one would pay the entire $79. Wouldn't it be worth asking their doctors about OTC alternatives regardless of insurance status? There are several reasons why doctors don't always tell you about OTCs, but the primary one is that there are 90,000 drug sales reps out there whose only purpose in life is to convince doctors to prescribe their particular drugs and to forget the very existence of OTC and generic meds—and it works. Most doctors will be relieved to hear you ask this question, so ask.

Question #3: Are there any generic meds that will do the job?
Potential Savings: 80–90%

We are currently in the midst of a flood of expensive brand name drugs losing their patents and going generic. As these drug formulas fall into the public domain, any qualified manufacturer can make and distribute these drugs, as long as it can meet the same stringent FDA quality standards as the original brand name version. This brings competition to a formerly monopoly-dominated market, and prices usually drop dramatically as a result—normally by 80–90% within the first year. Virtually every major class of drugs now has, or soon will have, a well-proven generic that works as well for most patients as its much more expensive branded cousins. Ask.

Question #4: If there are no OTCs or generics, can you prescribe the lowest priced brand name drug that will meet my needs?
Potential Savings: 40%

There's a well-kept secret in the pharmaceutical business that, within a given class of medications, equivalent but different brand name drugs can have big differences in price. When this is the case—and when there is no equivalent generic—you want your doctor to prescribe the lowest cost brand that will work for you. For example, Protonix costs significantly less than Nexium, but works as well for most patients with heartburn. Doctors will be frequently stumped by this particular question (although pharmacists won't), but ask it anyway. If they hear the question enough, they'll start to learn the answers.

Question #5: Can you prescribe a pill-splitting dose?
Potential Savings: 30–50%

If the medication your doctor is prescribing comes in tablet form, your doctor may be able to prescribe a double-strength tablet and then have you take a half tablet at a time. Often, the double-strength pill costs virtually the same as the smaller one, so you can save up to 50% with this technique. Many tablets are already scored with a groove across the middle to facilitate splitting with just your hands. But you can also buy a little guillotine-like pill-splitter from any drugstore for a few dollars to use for un-scored pills. (I sometimes use scissors.) This technique isn't appropriate for all drugs or all patients, but when it is, it saves a lot of money. Doctors are quite familiar with this approach, having been writing pill-splitting prescriptions for the elderly (to save money) and for children (to reduce doses) for a long time. Ask.

Question #6: For my maintenance medications, would you please write two prescriptions: one for a 30-day supply and another for a refillable 90-day or 100-day supply so I can buy from a mail-service pharmacy?
Potential Savings: 15–60%

If you know for sure that a maintenance drug does work for you, then mail service pharmacies can save you a lot of money. If you're paying the entire bill, then surfing the Web for high-quality, low-cost American pharmacies is worth the modest effort. If you have insurance coverage, most companies let you buy 90-day supplies for home delivery for lower copayments than you would have to pay at retail; and sometimes you can actually find the same drugs online for less than even the copayment—especially generic drugs. Just make sure that the drug works for you before asking for large quantities. Otherwise, you could be stuck with a large supply of useless pills. That's why you should ask for a 30-day Rx to buy locally, so you can find out if it works. Better yet, if your doctor can get you started on free samples (but *only* if there are no OTC or generic drugs), then you can forego the

30-day Rx altogether and save even more. Once you know that the drug works, use the 90-day or 100-day Rx to buy from a home-delivery pharmacy.

Question #7: May I please have a lot of extra samples of any brand name drugs you prescribe?
Potential Savings: 10–15%

Tell your doctor you have to pay for your own drugs, and ask if he can give you extra samples. Depending on how well supplied he is at the time, he may give you as much as a 30-day supply of drugs every visit at no charge, thus cutting your annual cost by 10–15%, or more. Just remember, you only want samples when there are no lower cost OTC or generic drugs available for your condition. Always ask, even when you're seeing a doctor for something else.

YOUR PHARMACIST IS AN ALLY, TOO

Whether or not you ask your doctor the 7 Questions, you can always get a second chance by asking the pharmacist the same questions. If your doctor has just given you samples and a prescription for 50 mg tablets of an expensive brand name drug to take once a day, ask your pharmacist how much it will cost if you were instead to take half of a daily 100 mg pill. Or ask if there are generic or over-the-counter drugs that do the same thing as the brand name. Ask her about what other doctors are prescribing for your condition. You will find that pharmacists have far more knowledge about medications than just how to count pills, and they are almost always happy to share that knowledge with you. Counting pills is a lot less professionally satisfying than counseling patients with their great depth of knowledge.

While the pharmacist cannot change your doctor's prescription on her own, she will almost certainly be willing to call your doctor on your behalf and ask if he would be willing to modify his original prescription in order to save you money. Pharmacists already spend a lot of time phoning doctors to change prescriptions written in error or not allowed by HMOs, so this won't be an imposition. In fact, it can be a welcome opportunity for the pharmacist to do something that the patient actually wants. And of course, if she won't do it, take your business elsewhere.

CHAPTER 5

What About Over-the-Counter Drugs?

Over-the-counter (OTC) drugs containing approximately 1000 active ingredients and used in more than 100,000 medications now account for about 60% of all drugs sold in the United States. Sales of these OTCs exceed $17 billion annually.[1, 2] These medications represent an inexpensive and effective first line of defense against approximately 400 different medical problems, and many are as effective as prescription drugs.

For example, the active ingredient in the antihistamine Benadryl is called diphenhydramine. Used to treat allergies, itching, cold symptoms, and insomnia, it is currently included in more than 100 brand name OTC drugs. Generic versions are even more numerous.[3]

Many people believe that OTC drugs can't possibly be as effective as prescription drugs, particularly the newer ones that we keep hearing cost $800 million or more to develop. In fact, many OTCs, including Benadryl,[4] were once highly effective prescription drugs that were switched to OTC status. OTC prices are usually a small fraction of those for the previous prescription versions.

Over the years, many safe, effective, and expensive prescription drugs have made the switch to over-the-counter as cheap, diagnose-yourself, go-down-to-the-supermarket-and-pluck-it-off-the-shelf drugs. While many are not in full prescription strength, your doctor may instruct you to take more than the labeled instructions indicate, thus giving you a full prescription dose of the medication. The OTC versions of such drugs as Claritin and Prilosec are the same strength they were as top-selling prescription meds. Overall, there are now more than 700 OTC products on the market that contain ingredients that required prescriptions twenty-five years ago.

The FDA itself had been a big proponent of Rx-to-OTC switches, with a stated goal of increasing the number making the change by 50%. Many OTC drugs have become household names, and we tend to forget that they were once available only by prescription. You will recognize some of the following:[5,6]

OTC Meds Previously Requiring a Prescription	
Heartburn	Prilosec
	Tagamet
	Pepcid
	Zantac
	Axid
Cold & Allergy	Claritin
	Loratadine

OTC Meds Previously Requiring a Prescription (cont'd)	
	Benadryl Tavist-1 NasalCrom
Diarrhea	Imodium Lomotil
Fungus Infection	Lotrimin Femstat Monistat
Hair Growth	Rogaine
Smoking Cessation	Nicorette NicoDerm Nicotrol
Pain & Inflammation	Advil Aleve Motrin Nuprin Orudis

Make no mistake. OTCs are powerful drugs. One particular medication available over-the-counter in the U.S., and in full strength, is arguably the greatest wonder drug of all time. It prevents strokes, reduces arthritis suffering, dampens inflammation, prevents heart attacks, reduces cancer risk, prevents vascular disease, and controls headaches—all for about half a cent per tablet. It can also cause serious side effects. It is, of course, aspirin. It has been suggested that if aspirin had been launched in 1999 instead of 1899, you'd now need a prescription to get it.[7]

Not every application to the FDA to switch status has been approved. Two notable recent rejections were for Mevacor (a statin drug for cholesterol control) and Plan B for postcoital pregnancy-prevention. Neither was considered by the FDA to be sufficiently safe or self-diagnosable for it to allow OTC status.

BEHIND THE COUNTER DISPENSING

Interestingly, Zocor, another statin similar to Mevacor, has been approved in Great Britain for over-the-counter sale, although the term has a different meaning there. In the U.S. over-the-counter really means off-the-shelf. You can walk into the store, take it off the shelf, pay for it, and consume it without ever having any professional screening or counseling. In Britain, over-the-counter really means behind-the-counter.[8] To buy it, you have to speak with a pharmacist who screens you for appropriateness of therapy and then counsels you about safe consumption and side effects. In the case of Zocor, British pharmacists (or chemists as they call them) confer with the consumer to determine that he is at moderate or high risk of heart disease, and then tells him how to spot symptoms of potentially dangerous muscle pains or liver disease before dispensing it. There is no equivalent behind-the-counter system in the United States, although sale of the common decongestant pseudoephedrine seems to migrating in that direction to prevent diversion of the drug into the illegal drug conversion market (the bad guys make methamphetamine from it).[9] Also, the New York legislature passed legislation in 2005 that would have allowed pharmacists to dispense Plan B from behind the counter, although the bill was vetoed by the governor.[10]

OTC DOUBLE COST ADVANTAGE

OTC medications carry two big cost advantages over prescription drugs. They have much lower price tags than prescription drugs, and you don't have to pay for a doctor to prescribe them.

OTC APPROVAL

Who determines whether a drug is to be prescription or OTC? Drug manufacturers have almost always asked that any new drugs be approved by the FDA as prescription rather than OTC drugs. They make a number of claims as to why that is, but there is no question that they can charge a far higher price for a prescription medication covered by insurance than for an OTC drug that isn't. Usually, you only see a prescription drug being converted to OTC when the patent on the Rx version runs out, thus exposing it to generic competition. Moving the drug to OTC can be a way for the manufacturer to continue to benefit from a drug's brand name that has received so much promotion and public recognition during its years as a prescription drug. Until recently, it was always the choice of the drug manufacturer whether to ask the

FDA for OTC approval for a drug. This changed dramatically in 2002 when WellPoint Health Networks, a health insurer, petitioned the FDA to approve several prescription-only antihistamines for OTC sale. The result was that the blockbuster drug Claritin and its generic siblings are now available OTC. Unfortunately, this activism by interested third parties has yet to become a trend, and Claritin remains the only OTC medication approved through this third party process.

The FDA holds final authority in these Rx/OTC switch decisions. In deciding whether to approve a switch application, the FDA asks four basic scientific and medical questions:[11]

1. Is there a low potential for abuse or misuse?
2. Can consumers use it for self-diagnosed conditions?
3. Can the drug be clearly and adequately labeled for consumers?
4. Can the drug be safely and effectively used without the need for doctors?

If the answer to all these questions is yes, then the FDA will usually allow the switch, but not always. In one of the most controversial decisions in recent memory, the FDA in 2004 rejected Plan B's application despite the overwhelming recommendation of the agency's own scientific advisers that the pregnancy prevention drug is safe and effective. Some suggest that politics may have been involved.[12]

OTC'S WEIRD ECONOMICS

Once a drug goes from being a prescription brand name to an OTC drug, the economics can get pretty strange. In general, the drug's price plunges, with the drugmaker achieving only about 10%[13] of the drug's former sales dollar volume. You would think that consumers would be the immediate winners in this deal. Oddly, they sometimes aren't. Take the case of Claritin, the monstrously successful prescription non-sedating antihistamine that became available as an OTC drug in late 2002. Prior to the switch, a month's supply of thirty tablets cost about $100.[14] Immediately afterward, it cost about $30.[15] Under the heading of no-good-deed-goes-unpunished, Claritin consumers were outraged at the change. It turns out that most of them were getting it under their health insurance plans for a monthly co-payment of about $15. But when the drug switched to OTC status, it was no longer a covered benefit, since only prescription drugs are usually covered by insurance. That meant that the patients now had to pay the full $30 retail price of the drug—a doubling of their cost! Fortunately, these aggrieved consumers can now buy generic Claritin (loratadine) for about $3 a month, so this particular problem was short-lived. But it does highlight how dumb a system is that makes a $30 drug look more expensive than a $100 one.

OTC DANGERS

We tend to forget that OTC drugs, taken incorrectly, can be just as dangerous as many Rx medications. Even when administered under a doctor's advice, it is always a good idea to read the product label for indications, dosing, and contraindications. Your doctor may specify a higher dose, however. If that concerns you, be sure to ask your doctor why. Without a doctor's advice, it is highly advisable to read and heed the labeled instructions and warnings. Unfortunately, the OTC drug manufacturers seem to have perfected the art of tiny, almost nanoscale printing that defies reading by all but the youngest eyes. It's not entirely their fault, since the FDA requires them to put so much information on the label that it is virtually impossible to do otherwise. If necessary, buy a magnifying glass, but do read the label. Death by side effect or overdose can be inconvenient.

HOW TO FIND THE RIGHT OTC MED

If you are currently seeing a doctor for a condition requiring prescription medications, I strongly urge you NOT to stop taking such drugs before getting your doctor's advice on switching to an OTC med.

When visiting your doctor for any condition, always ask if there are OTC alternatives to treat your condition. Don't assume he'll volunteer such information without being asked.

If you don't want to spend the time and money to see a doctor for your problem, the best personal source of information on OTC alternatives is your friendly, local pharmacist. Just make sure you're speaking with a pharmacist and not a pharmacy technician. Most pharmacies now have private consultation areas where you can speak without fear of being overheard by other shoppers. Describe your symptoms, and ask if there is a good OTC drug for your malady. Chances are that she'll come out from behind the counter, escort you to the proper aisle and shelf, and take down a bottle or box of something she recommends. If it's a brand name medication, ask if there is an identical but cheaper generic or store-brand—there usually is.

You can also find exhaustive information on OTC meds on the Internet, but beware of the mass of unreliable sites that can mislead you with crackpot or heavily biased information. Stick with sites that offer independent, science-based information. Useful sites include the following.

- **PDRhealth** at www.pdrhealth.com. A consumer-friendly guide to prescription drugs, OTC medications, herbal medicines, and nutritional supplements. Doctors use the professional version of the PDR (Physician's Desk Reference) daily to review drugs before prescribing for their patients. This website is produced by the same folks, but in patient-friendly layman's language. It's a wealth of information.
- **Costco** at www.costco.com. Not only does this commercial retail site offer useful information on all manner of OTC and prescription medication, it also offers some of the lowest prices I've seen for larger quantities of OTC meds. Just click on the "Pharmacy" button.
- **Hyde Rx** at www.hyderx.com. On my own website, you can find direct links to the above sites, as well as others that offer current information and prices on OTC and prescription meds.

CONCLUSION

Over-the-counter meds represent a huge opportunity for many patients to alleviate medical problems at very low cost. Don't hesitate to ask your doctor or pharmacist about them or to do your own homework. By definition, OTC drugs are intended for people who are capable of self-diagnosing and treating their own problems with little risk. Just be sure to read the labels, follow the directions, and heed the risks.

CHAPTER 6

What About Dietary Supplements and Herbal Medications?

Dietary supplements are hugely popular. I use the term to include complementary and alternative medicines, traditional remedies, herbal remedies, and dietary supplements of all sorts. All such products can be purchased off-the-shelf and are often sold directly by naturopaths, chiropractors, acupuncturists, and other practitioners. American consumers spend $30 billion a year of their own money on such treatments—about as much as they spend on medical doctors. According to a recent survey, nearly half of all online health information browsers who have disabilities or chronic diseases have searched online for information on dietary supplements and alternative treatments.[1]

For many people, dietary supplements offer relief from their medical problems. Many others are victimized by quacks and snake-oil salesmen selling useless nostrums that, at best, produce expensive urine, and, at worst, cause definite harm or lead the patient away from effective, critically necessary treatments. There is no area in health care where the advice caveat emptor is more appropriate. Unwary buyers can end up both sicker and poorer.

As with FDA-approved OTC medications, dietary supplements can offer a double dose of savings. Consumers can usually, but not always, buy them for much less than the cost of prescription drugs, and they don't have to pay a doctor to get them. The major difference is that dietary supplements, by definition, are *not* FDA-approved as safe and effective. In fact, they aren't regulated as drugs at all. More on that later.

FREQUENTLY TREATED CONDITIONS

Dietary supplements are most frequently sought for a wide variety of medical problems, including:[2]

- Back problems
- Allergies
- Arthritis
- Insomnia
- Sprains/strains
- Headaches
- High blood pressure
- Digestive problems
- Anxiety
- Depression
- Premenopausal symptoms

THREE CATEGORIES OF DIETARY SUPPLEMENTS

I find it useful to think about any dietary supplement as falling into one of three categories:

Category One products are those that have been scientifically shown to work safely and effectively in proper doses. Example: ginger for nausea prevention.

Category Two products are those that haven't been scientifically proven to be effective, but are still believed to be both safe and effective by many practitioners and consumers. Example: ginkgo biloba for memory improvement.

Category Three products are those that may or may not work, but have been found to be dangerous and sometimes fatal. Example: anabolic steroids for improved athletic performance.

There are relatively few Category One products, because there have been relatively few studies to scientifically establish them to be safe and effective. However, mushrooming interest in the category is spawning increased efforts by the U.S. government's Department of Agriculture and National Institutes of Health Office of Dietary Supplements and by independent nonprofit organizations to conduct the necessary scientific research to add to this list. For example, a search of the Office of Dietary Supplements' CARDS database of research projects on dietary supplements revealed 260 different in-process scientific studies on the effects of Vitamin E on a multitude of conditions and biologic processes.

The list of Category Two products is huge and fraught with uncertainty about effectiveness, safety, proper dosages, toxicity, active ingredient purity, pill-strength variations, and interactions with prescription and other medications. This category includes a lot of suspicious claims, con men and women, and outright fraud. It also includes medicines that have been used and believed to be safe and effective for hundreds of years. The problem, of course, is to be able to tell which is which.

Category Three products are those that have been found to injure or kill, but, unlike those in Categories One and Two, are subject to some regulation by the FDA. Unfortunately, the primary way to sort out Category Three dietary supplements is to retrospectively identify members of the public who have been harmed or killed by consuming such products. Unlike prescription and OTC drugs, there is no required testing for safety or efficacy before these products are marketed.

LIMITED REGULATION

Dietary supplements are not regulated as drugs as a result of the 1994 Dietary Supplement Health and Education Act (DSHEA). This federal law allows dietary supplements to bear claims that the products affect structures or functions of the human body, but they cannot claim to prevent, treat, or cure disease. That's why saw palmetto extract is sold "to promote prostate health" instead of "to prevent prostate cancer." There is no requirement to list inactive ingredients on the label, or even to list the product with the FDA. The FDA's role is effectively limited to identifying and pulling unsafe alternative medications from the market. Further confusing the regulatory environment is the fact that the FTC (Federal Trade Commission) is separately responsible for regulating dietary supplement advertising and for stopping false claims.

The DSHEA requires the following labeling requirements for dietary supplements:[3]

- Identity (e.g., saw palmetto)
- Net quantity (e.g., number of capsules)
- Active ingredients and amounts
- Disclaimer: "This statement has not been evaluated by the Food and Drug Administration. This product is not intended to diagnose, treat, cure, or prevent any disease."
- Directions for use
- Supplement facts panel, which includes serving size, amount, and active ingredient
- Other ingredients for which no daily value has been established
- Name and address of manufacturer, packer, or distributor

Essentially, as long as a manufacturer doesn't call its product a drug and doesn't claim it can prevent, treat, or cure disease, it can often get by with making completely unsubstantiated claims about its health-giving benefits. Let me say this again: if ever there was a let-the-buyer-beware category of products, this one is it.

LACK OF MANUFACTURER RESEARCH

Alternative medicines are rarely patented or patentable, so virtually anyone can make them as generic products that can be sold over-the-counter. Many such products are marketed under trademarked brand names, but the ingredients themselves are not patented. Because of the lack of manufacturing exclusivity, there is no incentive for manufacturers to conduct expensive, controlled trials to determine the true effectiveness and safety of their products. It is easier and more profitable to ride the rising current of popular enthusiasm for over-the-counter "natural" remedies.

MEDICAL DOCTORS GETTING INVOLVED

The increased credibility and popularity of the category has resulted in an increasing number of mainstream medical providers offering alternative and complementary products and services in concert with more traditional American-style allopathic medicine. This combined approach is often called "integrative" medicine.

One problem noted by many doctors is the estimated two-thirds of all patients who fail to list their alternative medicines and dietary supplements among the medications they take when responding to doctors' or druggists' questions about current medications.[4] This may arise from the ambiguous nature of dietary supplements, or a simple concern by patients that their doctors will disapprove of them. However, this information can be critical in identifying the potential for unwanted effects or harmful interactions with prescription drugs. For example, use of the popular dietary supplement echinacea for an extended period of time can cause elevation of liver enzymes, and people with certain conditions such as multiple sclerosis should not take it at all. The active ingredient in the natural product Saint-John's-wort can react negatively with antidepressants, alcohol, and certain foods. Ginseng root extracts have been linked with high blood pressure and irregular heartbeat problems. Ephedra, a naturally occurring botanical substance taken for weight loss, has been associated with death.

It should be apparent that, just because a product is marketed as "natural," it isn't necessarily safe. Nature is eminently capable of producing poisons and toxic substances. While you don't have to have your doctor's permission to take alternative remedies, you do have an obligation to her and to yourself to tell her about any such meds you're taking during a medical visit whether she asks the question or not. Otherwise, she might unwittingly prescribe something that can interact dangerously with them.

Three good rules to follow:

1. **Know what you're taking.** Do your own homework about alternative medicines, and be prepared to take responsibility for your failures as well as successes.

2. **Look for quality products.** Purchase only dietary supplements containing the USP mark on the label. This certifies that the United States Pharmacopeia company has tested and verified that it contains the stated ingredients in the declared amounts, that it has been screened for harmful contaminants, that it was made according to good manufacturing practices, and

that it will dissolve appropriately to release its active ingredients into your body. This does not certify that the product is either safe or effective, however, so Rule 1 still applies.

3. **Tell your doctor.** Most doctors will have you fill out a form listing any medications you are currently taking, and many will also have their nurses ask this question directly. Be sure to reveal any dietary supplements, natural remedies, or alternative medicines that you are taking, whether the question is asked or not. If your doctor disapproves in principle, but you are strongly inclined toward alternative medicine, then look for a different doctor who is more attuned to your attitude. Having a doctor you don't respect or won't heed is not a good situation for either of you.

In the homework category, there are numerous websites providing information on alternative medicines, but most of them are either blatantly or secretly commercial and offer little in the way of unbiased information. However, several websites do report independent, unbiased, noncommercial information that can be very useful to patients. Here are some sites that I've found to be particularly helpful. You can also check my website (www.HydeRx.com) for updated links.

M. D. Anderson Cancer Center

http://www.mdanderson.org/departments/cimer/din dex.cfm?pn = 6eb86a59-ebd9-11d4-810100508b603- a14

Entering this terribly complicated Web address in your browser will ironically yield one of the more accessible and comprehensive sources of current information on a wide range of alternative, complementary, and integrative therapies (you can also just enter www.mdanderson.org, but you'll have to do some further navigation once you're there). The website is maintained by the prestigious University of Texas M.D. Anderson Cancer Center and covers many therapies other than just cancer-related ones.

Memorial Sloan-Kettering Cancer Center

http://www.mskcc.org/mskcc/html/11570.cfm
An encyclopedic, but more technical site from Memorial Sloan-Kettering Cancer Center with information on many alternative therapies.

National Center for Complementary and Alternative Medicine (National Institutes of Health)

http://nccam.nih.gov/clinicaltrials/treatment therapy.htm
If you're interested in participating in a clinical trial of alternative therapies, or if you just want to know the current state of scientific research, this website by the National Center for Complementary and Alternative Medicine lists more than eighty trials currently recruiting patients or under way.

MedlinePlus (National Institutes of Health)

http://www.nlm.nih.gov/medlineplus/complemen taryandalternativetherapies.html
This site by the National Institutes of Health's MedlinePlus is a useful clearinghouse for information on herbal treatments for different medical conditions.

Quackwatch.org

www.quackwatch.org

This site administers a strong dose of sunlight to many of the darker corners of alternative therapy. It is maintained by Stephen Barrett, MD, a retired psychiatrist, and makes for fascinating reading.

THE ULTIMATE SUPER DRUG—PLACEBOS

Placebos are sugar pills given to control-group patients in experimental drug trials to see how they respond when compared to patients who have taken the actual medication being tested. Neither the control patients nor the test subjects know which pill they're getting, and usually the doctors administering the tests don't know, either.

A couple of years ago, a brand name drug company ran an advertisement with a chart showing how effective two of its drugs were in treating major depression. The chart showed how the two medications used in an actual clinical trial, Celexa and Lexapro, affected major depression in the participants. The part that's so fascinating is not that the two tested medications actually worked, but that a placebo worked almost as well as the drugs. The real drugs improved patients' conditions by about thirteen points on the chart's scale, while the placebo group had an improvement of almost ten points.

One might reasonably expect the placebo patients to respond no differently from patients given no treatment at all, but that's not how it works out. In fact, patients on placebo have shown remarkable improvement for conditions such as high blood pressure, depression, asthma, allergies, pain (including angina), gastric reflux disease, and even Parkinson's disease. One wag has suggested that the only problem with this is that placebos also have side effects, such as high blood pressure, depression, asthma, allergies, etc.[5]

Placebos have been surprisingly effective for many maladies. I sometimes wonder why the sugar companies haven't marketed the stuff as a miracle dietary supplement. Seriously, the key seems to be that the placebo patient actually believes he will get better, which somehow results in his body beginning to actively and effectively mount its own unconscious, largely unknown healing defenses—a process I call autonomic healing. In one such test, doctors in Toronto administered either fluoxetine (the generic drug formerly known as Prozac) or a placebo to seventeen depressed men.[6] Of the ten men receiving the actual drug, four improved. Of the seven receiving the placebo, four improved. When the men on placebo were told the truth, all but one relapsed into depression. Interestingly, the one who didn't relapse realized he could stay better on his own—and did.

This raises the question of whether you can put the placebo effect to work for you. Theoretically, that would be the cheapest medication ever. It should be obvious that popping M&M's won't do you any good (make that any "clinical" good), since there's no earthly reason for you to believe there is any real drug in there. And no doctor is going to prescribe sugar pills and tell you they're a miracle drug, lest he be found guilty of malpractice.

Maybe there is a way to try it, though. The technique I have in mind involves taking one of those OTC herbal or alternative remedies that you believe will work. You can easily check out the above Internet sites that will give you information on how such remedies may be able to prevent, alleviate, or cure what-ever disease you may be concerned with.

If you see something promising *and safe*—even if there is no particular scientific basis for the sub-stance's therapeutic effectiveness—then you can give it a try. The key is that you actually believe it will work. If it does, then terrific. The thing is, you won't really know whether it's because the product is actually bioactively dealing with your problem or whether it's because of autonomic healing. Nor should you care, as long as it's actually working. But if it doesn't work, then you have only created expensive body waste, as-suming you don't have any adverse reactions.

Just be aware that it is unlikely that most such reme-dies will ever be tested to the extent necessary to satisfy the FDA of their actual safety and efficacy. *In no event should you stop taking any currently prescribed drugs without first talking to your doctor.* And make sure—by asking your doctor, asking your pharmacist, or doing your own homework—that the "placebo" you decide to try isn't dangerous and won't interfere or negatively in-teract with your prescription or OTC medications.

CHEAPER

This a book about getting the drugs you need at the low-est possible cost. Legitimate dietary supplements can fit into this scenario if (1) you buy something that really works; and (2) you don't spend more than you would have for an equivalent prescription drug, if there is one.

As I've already discussed, finding what you need in a field with so little comparative scientific information can make finding the right preparation a hit-or-miss proposition. When you do find something that works, and it happens to be a proprietary product, then it can be difficult or impossible to find generic equivalent formulations of the same stuff at a lower price. On the other hand, you can find multiple versions of standard preparations of an increasing number of single-ingredient or standard-combination dietary supplements, such as vitamins, mineral supplements, ginkgo biloba, echinacea, glucosamine with chondroitin, and many others. Such products are as close as you'll find to generic equivalents in the dietary supplement world.

Many consumers buy their dietary supplements from their healthcare providers. In fact the sale of such products seems to constitute a significant part of the revenue of chiropractors, acupuncturists, naturopaths, and other alternative healthcare providers. Obtaining a product from a trained and certified practitioner can go a long way toward assuring you of its safety and efficacy. It can also be an expensive way to buy it, however, as these practitioners often charge higher prices than stores.

Medical doctors have largely moved away from dispensing and selling drugs to their patients, with notable exceptions for cancer drugs and injectables. Among other issues, there are ethical concerns about a doctor prescribing a drug from which he makes a profit, which may create an incentive for the doctor to prescribe more than you need. When I was in the medical group management business, I noticed a huge difference between the number of lab tests ordered by doctors depending on whether they received a portion of the test revenue or not. Those who did were much higher utilizers of such tests. The same incentives hold for doctors and practitioners who sell drugs or related products. This is one area where medical doctors are increasingly at variance with alternative practitioners.

If you buy from a practitioner and you are satisfied with the product, you are under no obligation to continue to obtain it from your care provider. Instead, you can seek alternate, lower cost sources, such as those discussed below.

When you do find a product that you like, finding it in a store at the lowest price can be a chore because many products are not widely distributed. You can use the same comparison-shopping techniques discussed in Chapter 11 to improve your chances, but it's not equivalent to calling several drugstores knowing that all of them are likely to have the product that you need. Your best route is the Internet. Let's say, for example, that you take the proprietary supplement Biolean Free Herbal & Amino Acid Dietary Supplement, and you want to pay as little as possible for it. You can fire up your computer and go to your favorite search engine website (e.g., www.turboscout.com, www.teoma.com, www.yahoo.com, or www.google.com) and enter the search words "Biolean Free Herbal & Amino Acid Dietary Supplement Wellness International price" (but without the quotation marks). When I did this on one search engine, I found 732 results that more or less matched my criteria. This demonstrates both the challenge and the opportunity of finding what you need on the Internet. On the one hand, the challenge is to sift through 732 sites to find the best deal. On the other, the opportunity rests in the fact that somewhere in those 732 sites *is* probably the best deal. I was able to do an advanced search with the same terms and narrow the number of hits to only 35. From these, I found prices ranging from $57.95 to $69.95 for a 28-day supply.

I then tried Yahoo!'s shopping site (http://shop ping.yahoo.com) and found it much easier to use than the above shotgun approach, and quickly located the

Biolean Free being sold at prices ranging from $53.00 to $69.95. I cannot vouch for the reputation of any of these (or any other) sellers, so that will add another layer of caveat emptor to your dietary supplement search. You may have heard the saying, "On the Internet, nobody knows you're a dog."

When searching on the Internet, it is important to refine your searches to get a manageable result. When I entered "gingko biloba price," the search engine returned 319,000 results! But when I entered, "Nature's Answer Ginkgo Leaf (Alcohol Free)", the engine returned "only" 5,860 matches. Yahoo! Shopping immediately found multiple sellers with prices from $5.75 to $9.66. Pretty cool service. There are entire books on how to optimize search engine use, but you don't have to read a book (except this one) to find what you need on the Web. If you run out of options like these to narrow your search, check out five or six of the most promising looking sites that want to sell you your stuff.

CONCLUSION

Dietary supplements are a booming business and offer relief to many thousands of consumers, often at prices below prescription drugs. Independent researchers are increasingly demonstrating the reliability with which an increasing number of these products and formulations can allow you to get the results you desire as reliably and as safely as you can in the prescription and OTC drug world. But the industry has a long way to go to achieve the assurances of safety and effectiveness offered by the regulated drug world. Trained practitioners can help you find the right products, and the Internet can help you get them at the lowest cost.

CHAPTER 7

Go Generic or Switch to Lower-Priced Brands

GENERIC DRUGS

Buying generic drugs represents the single most effective way most patients can get the drugs they need at the lowest possible cost. According to data from the National Association of Chain Drug Stores, the average 2004 price for a generic prescription was $28.74, compared to the average brand prescription at $96.01.[1] Actually, this generic price considerably overstates how much a savvy shopper can actually pay, as generics are not only the best bargain in health care, they are the most marked-up drugs on the market. Careful comparison shoppers will usually pay about half this average (see Chapter 11). Not only are generics just as good as the brands they replace, but we're now seeing a lot more of them.

We are in the midst of a revolution in the availability of cheap, powerful, generic prescription drugs. From 2002 through 2006 alone, brand name drugs with more than $20 billion in annual sales will have lost their twenty-year patent protection (see table below), opening them to generic competition. This means that a multitude of generic drug manufacturers will be able to produce cheap, high quality copies of what had once been expensive brand name drugs. If recent history is a guide, within the first year of generic competition, the cost of these copies will be *80–90% lower* than the brand name drugs they replace.

Your challenges will be (1) to overcome massive promotion and manipulation by the brand name drug industry to keep you away from generics, and (2) to buy them without having to pay huge markups. I'll tell you how to do both.

Twelve Major Brand Name Drug Patent Expirations				
2000 Sales in Billions of Dollars				
Brand	**Indication**	**Expiration**	**Patent Holder**	**2000 Sales (b$)**
Prilosec (omeprazole)	Heartburn, ulcer	2003	Astra Zeneca	4.1
Prevacid (lansoprazole)	Heartburn, ulcer	2005	Tap Pharma	2.8
Zocor (simvastatin)	Cholesterol	2005	Merck	2.2
Zoloft (sertraline)	Depression	2005	Pfizer	1.9

Twelve Major Brand Name Drug Patent Expirations (cont'd)

2000 Sales in Billions of Dollars

Brand	Indication	Expiration	Patent Holder	2000 Sales (b$)
Paxil (paroxetine)	Depression	2006	Glaxo Smith Kline	1.8
Claritin (loratadine)	Allergy	2002	Schering-Plough	1.7
Pravachol (pravastatin)	Cholesterol	2005	Bristol-Myers Squibb	1.2
Neurontin (gabapentin)	Epilepsy	2002	Pfizer	1.1
Cipro (ciprofloxacin)	Infection	2003	Bayer	1.0
Zestril (lisinopril)	Hypertension	2002	Astra Zeneca	0.8
Singulair (montelukast)	Asthma	2003	Merck	0.7
Flovent (fluticasone)	Asthma	2003	Glaxo Smith Kline	0.6

Source: Generic Pharmaceutical Association

The blockbuster conversions listed above are only the barest tip of the iceberg. There are thousands of proven generic drugs to treat hundreds of diseases and conditions. Appendix E lists many common conditions, along with a variety of OTC, generic, and lower cost brand name drugs that are currently available to treat them. Appendix F provides a longer list of recent and upcoming brand name drug patent expirations.

If you want to find out if any of your brand name drugs are nearing generic status, the FDA operates a useful, if rather technical, website at http://www.fda.gov/cder/ogd/approvals/default.htm. It is not particularly easy for the layman to follow, but it lists generic approvals by month of approval, and shows them in three categories:

1. "Approvals" of any new generics
2. "First Generics" for drugs never before approved as generic drugs
3. "Tentative Approvals" for drugs pending patent expiration

Another useful FDA site is the Electronic Orange Book (http://www.fda.gov/cder/ob/default.htm). You can't miss it—it's salmon pink (go figure). You can enter a drug by brand name or by the active ingredient (i.e., the generic name), and it will show you any approved generic drugs.

A more accessible website to determine if your drug is available generically is operated by the state of North Dakota at http://governor.state.nd.us/pharmaceutical/. This site, however, is not as up-to-date as the FDA site.

Websites are continually arriving, departing, or changing URL addresses. I maintain current linkages to the ones I find most useful at www.HydeRx.com.

Unfortunately, you cannot assume that your doctor will automatically prescribe a generic drug for you, assuming one is available. Most doctors aren't even aware that a new generic has become available. Instead, he will usually give you a bunch of free samples and a written prescription for a much more expensive brand name drug. You can thank the brand name drug companies for this. They are putting their money, might, and manpower behind an effort to keep you, your doctor, and your insurance company (if you're lucky enough to have one) focused on newer, ever-more-expensive brand name drugs that may be no better for you than available generics.

ARE GENERIC DRUGS REALLY AS GOOD AS BRANDS?

According to the Food and Drug Administration (FDA), generic drugs are every bit as good as their brand name equivalents, and they are fully interchangeable. Says Gary Buehler, director of FDA's Office of Generic Drugs, "Most people believe that if something costs more it has to be better quality. In the case of generic drugs, this is not true. People can use them with total confidence."[2] The FDA requires all generic drugs to have the same quality, effectiveness, strength, safety, bioequivalence, purity, solubility, and stability as brand name drugs. And not only are generic drugs manufactured in plants meeting the same quality standards as those making brand name drugs, but an estimated half of all generic drugs are actually manufactured by brand name firms.

The FDA regularly tests generic drugs to evaluate

their conformance with these standards, and it unequivocally states, "To date, there are no documented examples of a generic product manufactured to meet its approved specifications that could not be used interchangeably with the corresponding brand-name drug."[3] Despite these assurances, many people, including a lot of doctors, still persist in the belief that generics are somehow inferior.

There is another possible explanation for concern about the quality of generic drugs: narrow therapeutic index drugs (NTIs). NTIs, also called narrow therapeutic range drugs, consist of a relatively small number of medications in which the margin between a minimum *effective* dose and a minimum *toxic* dose is very small. Small changes in dosage and/or blood concentration of these drugs can cause problems of either inadequate treatment on the one hand or toxicity on the other.[4] Many doctors believe they will minimize any unwanted variation in drug dosage if they always specify only the brand name drugs in this category. These doctors will usually specify on the prescription "Brand Medically Necessary" and "Dispense as Written." That tells the pharmacist (and the insurance company) that generic substitution is *not* permitted for medical reasons.

There are relatively few drugs with NTIs, which are used primarily to treat stroke, asthma, epilepsy, hypertension, and other diseases requiring doctors to closely monitor and adjust doses. They include the following drugs (note: brands are capitalized and generics are lowercased and in parentheses):

- Tegretol (carbamazepine)
- Lanoxin (digoxin)

- Levothroid, Levoxyl, Synthroid, Unithroid (levothyroxine)
- Eskalith, Lithobid (lithium)
- Dilantin (phenytoin)
- Uniphyl, Theo-Dur (theophylline)
- Coumadin (warfarin)
- Duraquin (quinadine)
- Pronestyl, Procan-SR, Procanbid (procainamide)

The only problem with the all-too-common practice of prescribing only branded NTI drugs is that it has no basis in scientific fact. The FDA often requires or recommends additional testing by generic manufacturers of NTIs in order "to give the practitioner and patient additional assurance of product quality and interchangeability."[5] In a letter to doctors, the FDA concludes, ". . . in the judgment of the FDA, products evaluated as therapeutically equivalent can be expected to have equivalent clinical effect whether the product is brand name or generic drug product."[6]

In other words, any generic drug is just as good as the original brand name drug, and the two are completely interchangeable. The message you can take away from this is that you always want to ask your doctor to prescribe a lower cost generic instead of a brand name drug. Just be aware that you may encounter resistance from your doctor regarding NTI generics, and in the end, your doctor must make the final decision on prescribing your drugs. Fortunately, NTI brands don't always cost all that much more than the generics.

HOW TO MISS OUT ON A NEW GENERIC DRUG

I've already written about how the brand name drug companies spend $15 billion a year promoting their expensive prescription products. A key part of this promotion is the "gift" of "free" samples of branded medications to virtually every doctor in America who is willing to take them. But when a drug nears its inevitable patent loss, all such promotional efforts cease, often in favor of a newer "improved" version of the soon-to-be-generic drug—the improvement is often either a time-release version of exactly the same active ingredient or a slightly altered molecule, either of which can result in a new, longer patent life.

For example, in 2002 Schering-Plough transferred its huge promotional efforts from its prescription antihistamine Claritin to its newer Clarinex, a very similar drug with similar results. Likewise, stomach acid blocker Prilosec was supplanted by Nexium; and antidepressant Celexa by Lexapro. Such replacements tend to offer few improvements over their predecessors for most patients. Indeed, Lexapro has actually been advertised as being "equivalent" to Celexa, the older drug.

In reviewing the history of many such promotional shifts to newer me-too drugs, I have identified eight steps that drug companies regularly follow in trying to get you to shift to more expensive drugs, when you could have simply stayed with an effective, time-tested brand that is about to become available generically at much lower cost.

1. **It's Been Fun, But . . .** In this first step, the current brand name drug (e.g., Claritin, Prilosec,

Celexa, Prozac, Allegra 60 mg, Glucophage) nears the end of its twenty-year exclusive patent protection period.

2. **New and Improved—More or Less ...** A year or two before the established drug's patent expires, the manufacturer introduces an "upgraded" version of the old drug with a longer remaining patent life (e.g., Clarinex, Nexium, Lexapro, Prozac Weekly, Allegra 180 mg, Glucophage XR). The new drug often offers only marginal benefit over the old one, and is often just an extended release formulation of the same active ingredient that may add some patient convenience, but little or nothing in the way of safety or efficacy. According to Marcia Angell, MD, the former editor of *The New England Journal of Medicine,* "78% of drugs approved by FDA in the past six years were classified as unlikely to be better than existing ones. 60% didn't even contain new active ingredients."[7]

3. **Alienation of Affections.** After introducing the me-too replacement, the manufacturer drops all advertising, promotion, rebates, and free samples of the older, established brand name drug version.

4. **Transfer of Affections.** The manufacturer then shifts all those resources and more, often amounting to hundreds of millions of dollars, to the new drug. On top of that, manufacturers have actually paid so-called switching fees to pharmacies and pharmacy benefit managers to reward them for successfully encouraging pa-

tients and their doctors to switch from the older, soon-to-be-cheap drug to the newer, will-continue-to-be-very-expensive drug. Thus, as you undoubtedly know if you've turned on a TV or opened a magazine or newspaper during the past year, Nexium is "the new purple pill" that, at $130 per month, or perhaps $25–35 per month if you have insurance, will cure your heartburn and make you smile, smile, smile. Do consumers or doctors remember that the old purple pill was Prilosec? Or know that Prilosec is now available over-the-counter in full prescription strength for about $17 per month (but now in salmon pink)? Or that Prilosec OTC works just as well as Nexium for most patients? Probably not.

5. **Younger AND Cheaper.** The manufacturer initially prices the new drug slightly lower than the older one in order to demonstrate a short-term savings for insurers and patients who switch. This step is very important, because it allows the drug companies to convince pharmacy benefit managers (PBMs), insurers, doctors, and their patients that not only is this drug newer and better (or at least newer), but it is also *cheaper*. Conveniently omitted from this sales point is that the old drug's soon-to-be-generic price is about to tumble by 80–90%. If the patients who were perfectly happy with the older drug just stayed on it, their savings on the generic version would be huge.

6. **The Switcheroo.** Doctors, insurance companies, and PBMs—led by the advertising, pro-

motion, rebates, free samples, switching fees, and general hype surrounding the new drug—encourage or even require patients to switch to the new version. The patient asks her doctor for the new drug she saw advertised on TV. The doctor is only too happy to respond with a prescription and a handful of free samples from the drug rep who just left after providing a free lunch for the entire office staff. The patient's employer or insurance company passively pays the lion's share of the drug's high price.

7. **Generic Who?** With the successful opening performance of the new medication, the older brand name drug finally, but quietly, goes generic with no promotion, no advertising, no drug reps, and with doctors' fading memory of its past greatness. And irony of ironies, the new generic drug isn't even very cheap. That's right, after all I've said about what a great bargain generics are, I now tell you that a brand new generic drug won't be—at least not initially. The reason is that the U.S. government, in its infinite special interest responsiveness, gives a six-month *monopoly* to the first generic manufacturer to successfully navigate the courts and the FDA to produce the first legal generic version of a brand name drug whose patent has expired. That's right. Just when you thought it was safe for the generic makers to enter the competitive waters, the drug police allow only one of them to jump into the pool.

They price it just enough lower than the equivalent brand, maybe 10% lower, to be able to show savings to the critics, but no more than necessary to take full advantage of many insurance companies' automatic policies of allowing coverage only for the generic version of any patent-expired brand name drug, rather than the brand itself. Only after the six month monopoly has expired—during which the generic manufacturer earns literally hundreds of millions in monopoly profits—does the market open up to the rest of the generic manufacturers, who pile in and compete on the only basis available to them, price. That's when you see the price drop, often by 80–90% during the ensuing six to twelve months.

But the hapless patient, who has long since been converted to the me-too brand replacement, sees none of these savings, even though the older drug worked just fine.

8. **Younger, Yes, but Just Kidding About Cheaper.** Remember Step 5 in which the new drug was priced cheaper than the old? Well, once the old drug has become available generically, this practice vanishes, and the drug company is free to raise the price on the new one for as long and as much as the market will bear. Usually, that means an increase of 6–10% per year, which is well in excess of the general inflation rate. Because most of the patients taking the drug have insurance and fixed-dollar rather than percentage copayments, they rarely see any of these price increases in a direct way. Instead, they see their copayments go up year after year on all their drugs, but nothing stands out about a particular drug. The problem with this, of course, is for folks like you who may have only limited

drug coverage—or no coverage at all. You bear the full brunt of these price increases.

As a result of this eight-step process, we have seen me-too brand drugs maximized, generics marginalized, and savings minimized. I may seem critical of the pharmaceutical manufacturers for such Machiavellian manipulations, but I would be hard-pressed to propose to them a better strategy for maximizing their profits under the current screwed up system of healthcare financing. While their executives may genuinely regret the impact on those innocent bystanders who lack comprehensive prescription drug insurance coverage, they are simply behaving rationally according to the rules of an irrational game. Until such time that the actual consumers—instead of their doctors—become the actual perceived cost-conscious customers for the drug manufacturers, this irrationality will remain and prescription drug prices will continue to outstrip the consumer price index.

BEWARE THE ME-TOO DRUG!

The above process of creating a new me-too drug to replace a new generic has been highly effective for many brand name drugmakers. But it has not always worked for some, as was the case with Lilly's replacement of Prozac with both Prozac Weekly and Serafem, both of which contain exactly the same active ingredient as Prozac. But that doesn't stop competing manufacturers of me-too drugs from stepping in and promoting *their* products as replacements for their soon-to-be-generic competitors. Thus, generic Prozac (fluoxetine) at $.10 a pill was largely supplanted by the brands Paxil, Zoloft, Celexa, and Lexapro at $2.50 or so per pill. It is true that these latter drugs often offer equivalent therapy with somewhat fewer unwanted side effects (and two of them, Paxil and Celexa, are now also available generically), but it is equally true that Prozac and its generic siblings continue to be just as safe and effective as when Prozac was one of the largest selling drugs in America, and most patients taking it do not experience such side effects. If it doesn't work the way the patient wants, he can go back to his doctor to consider alternatives.

The best way for you to opt out of drug company manipulation is to be knowledgeable about the drugs you take and the alternatives that are available. If you are taking a brand name drug that is about to be available as a generic, do not assume you will automatically be switched to the lower cost version by your doctor.

Besides the websites listed throughout this book, a good source of information is my website, www.HydeRx.com.

GENERIC DRUG PRICES

Which brings me to the subject of generic drug prices. I have gone on and on (and on) about how effective, safe, and cheap they are. But if all you do is walk into a drugstore and get your prescription filled for their cash price, you will likely be paying more than you need to—a lot more. This is also true of many mail order pharmacies.

The little-known secret of generic drugs is that they can be marked up from three to ten *times* their wholesale cost by the pharmacy, and yet still represent a savings over equivalent brand name drugs. For many pharmacies, generic drugs provide the highest profit margin—significantly higher than for brand name drugs.

When you get any prescription filled at retail, your price actually consists of two components, one is the ingredient cost of the drugs (i.e. the pills themselves), and the other is the professional dispensing fee charged by the pharmacist for filling the prescription. Thus, the drugstore can make money from both the markup on the drugs and the professional dispensing fee. For a variety of reasons, brand name drug margins tend to be skinny, but generic drugs offer significant opportunity for profit.

That is why comparison-shopping is so important in buying generic drugs. Read Chapter 11: "Savvy Shopping: Getting the Best Deal from Retail, Mail Order, and Internet Pharmacies." There I will tell you how to find pharmacies with the lowest prices.

WHAT'S THE DIFFERENCE BETWEEN A GENERIC EQUIVALENT DRUG AND A THERAPEUTICALLY SIMILAR DRUG?

It is important to make the distinction between generic equivalent drugs and therapeutically similar drugs, although I may be about to tell you more than you think you need to know. Trust me; this is important.

A *generic equivalent drug* is one with the same active chemical ingredient as its brand name original. A *therapeutically similar drug* is one which has a different chemical composition for its active ingredient from a specific brand name drug, but which nonetheless has a similar therapeutic effect for the condition being treated. To confuse matters further, a therapeutically similar drug may be either a generic or a brand name drug.

An example of two *generic equivalent drugs* is omeprazole (generic) and Prilosec (brand). The active, generic ingredient in each has exactly the same chemical structure and content, which is called omeprazole. Taking generic omeprazole is as good as taking brand name Prilosec (in the same dosage), since Prilosec is just omeprazole with a fancy, more expensive name. One is the same as the other with respect to its active ingredient, and both are interchangeable—and are thus generic equivalent drugs.

An example of two *therapeutically similar drugs* would be Prilosec and Protonix. Both are brand name drugs that are members of the same drug class—proton pump inhibitors, or PPIs. Both work on the same biochemical processes in the human body to suppress the secretion of stomach acid that contributes to heartburn, acid reflux disease, and stomach ulcers. But the active ingredient in Prilosec, again, is omeprazole, while the active ingredient in Protonix is pantoprazole, a different drug, but one which is in the same chemical class and works similarly to omeprazole. Thus, while they are therapeutically similar, they are *not* generically equivalent, because they have different chemical structures. Thus, they are not automatically interchangeable, although you may find you get the same therapeutic effect from one as the other.

Other therapeutically similar PPIs include Nexium, Aciphex, and Prevacid, each with its own active ingredient that is unique, but similar to that of the others. The medical use and outcomes are usually the same, so they are considered therapeutically similar drugs.

But because they do have different active ingredients, these drugs may sometimes have different effects in different people. While most people can take any of these PPIs with similar effect, some people may get better results from one than another.

Who cares? And do you really need to understand all this? The answers are: "You should," and "Yes," respectively. Here's why. Lots of times, your doctor may be inclined to prescribe a drug such as Lipitor. When you ask about generic drugs (Question #3), your doctor may say something like, "No, Lipitor is not available as a generic," and leave it at that. His answer is literally true because Lipitor's active ingredient, atorvastatin, is still covered by a patent until 2010 that prevents anyone but Pfizer from making and selling it.[4] However, you want your doctor to view the question more broadly, so that his answer is something like this, "Well, Lipitor is not available generically, but there is a drug that is therapeutically similar to it and works just as well for many patients requiring a 25–30% LDL cholesterol reduction. It's called lovastatin and is available generically. I could try putting you on that." Then you're talking about saving real money while getting, in this case, your LDL cholesterol lowered just as effectively by a therapeutically similar drug.

LOWER COST BRANDS

Even when a generic drug may not be available or the best choice for your condition, you may find there is a lower cost therapeutically similar brand name drug

Drug Classes by Cost

Drug Class	Treats	Generics (Brand Equivalent)	Lower Cost Brands	Other Brands
NSAs (non-steroidal anti-inflammatory)	Allergies	fexofenadine (Allegra), loratadine (OTC Claritin)	Zyrtec*	Allegra 180 mg Clarinex, Semprex
Statins	Cholesterol	lovastatin (Mevacor)	Lipitor, Crestor	Zocor, Pravachol
SSRIs (selective serotonin reuptake inhibitors)	Depression Anxiety	fluoxetine (Prozac), paroxetine (Paxil), citalopram (Celexa)	Lexapro	Luvox, Zoloft
ACE Inhibitors (angiotensin-converting enzyme inhibitors)	High Blood Pressure	captopril (Capoten), enalapril (Vasotec), lisinopril (Prinivil, Zestril)	Lotensin, Mavik, Univasc, Accupril	Aceon, Altace, Monopril
ARBs (angiotensin receptor blockers)	High Blood Pressure	N/A	Benicar, Teveten	Atacand, Avapro, Cozaar, Diovan, Micardis

Drug Classes by Cost (cont'd)

Drug Class	Treats	Generics (Brand Equivalent)	Lower Cost Brands	Other Brands
PPIs (proton pump inhibitors)	Stomach Acid Reflux, Ulcers	omeprazole (Prilosec)**	Prilosec OTC**, Protonix***	Nexium, AcipHex, Prevacid
NSAIDs (non-steroidal anti-inflammatory drugs)	Pain, Inflammation	diclofenac (Voltaren), ibuprofen (Advil, Motrin, Nuprin), naproxen (Aleve)	Mobic	Celebrex
TZDs (thiazolidinediones)	Diabetes	N/A	Avandia	Actos

*Although many doctors prescribe Zyrtec, it is not labeled as non-sedating.
**Generic prescription omeprazole and Prilosec OTC (available over the counter) have the same active ingredient. At the time of this writing, prescription omeprazole is approximately three to four times more expensive than Prilosec OTC *in the same 20 mg dose.* Whenever possible, ask your doctor to prescribe or recommend Prilosec OTC instead of generic omeprazole.
***Protonix is generally 20% less expensive than Nexium, AcipHex, or Prevacid, but is still about five times more expensive than Prilosec OTC for equivalent therapeutic effect for most patients.

that will work just as well as the more expensive one. Lipitor is a prime example. Not only is it the largest selling drug in the world, it is more effective at reducing LDL cholesterol and less expensive than most of the other brand name drugs in the statin class, such as Zocor and Pravachol.

The preceding are some of the major drug classes that have multiple drugs, along with the lower-priced drugs in each class.

ASK FOR STEP THERAPY

A good rule of thumb is to ask your doctor to start you on the least expensive therapeutically effective drug. If the results are unsatisfactory (inadequate effectiveness or unacceptable side effects) she may then change your prescription to the next higher cost drug, and so on. In the insurance trade, this is called *step therapy*, and your doctor will most likely be familiar with it and be willing to help you with it—if you ask. Your goal is to always get the drug you need, but at the lowest possible price. Let's face it; you don't really want the Nexium you've seen advertised interminably on TV. You want relief from your acid reflux–induced heartburn, and you want it to be cheap. Most of the time, that may mean taking Prilosec OTC (about $15–20 per month) instead of Nexium (about $130 per month if you're uninsured and probably $25–35 in copayments if you have insurance).

CONCLUSION

Generic drugs represent the best bargain in health care, but you may have to stay on your toes to get them. The brand name drug companies are very accomplished at getting patients to change drugs before a generic becomes available. You can work with your doctor to make sure this does not happen.

In cases where generics may not be available or effective, be sure to ask your doctor or pharmacist about lower cost brands. The United States healthcare system is probably the only industry in the country where a leading company can bring out a product that is equivalent to an established one, price it substantially higher, and still sell billions of dollars worth of the stuff.

PART III:

BUYING SOLUTIONS

Nobody wants to spend more money for prescription drugs than they have to. I have told you how to work with your doctor and your pharmacist to make sure that you always get prescriptions for the lowest cost medications that will meet your health care needs. Now I'm going to tell you about how to pay the lowest price for those drugs when you actually purchase them. Unfortunately, it is rarely a matter of simply taking those prescriptions to your local pharmacy and paying what they ask. Instead, there are a variety of ways for you to reduce your costs even further—often to zero for many people.

In the remainder of this book I will talk about drug purchase strategies. There are many options, including numerous free and discount drug programs as well as finding pharmacies offering the lowest prices. Once you have learned these techniques, you will be fully armed to get the drugs you need at the lowest cost.

One resource that you should know about is my website at www.HydeRx.com. Feel free to use it any time to help you locate low-cost pharmacies, identify free and discount drug programs, and stay current on low cost generic and OTC alternatives to expensive brand name drugs. This website is also a good way for you to give me feedback on how I can do a better job helping you to get the drugs you need at the lowest possible cost.

CHAPTER 8

Split Your Pills—
and Costs—in Half

Do you or anyone in your family take any of the prescription drugs in the table at the end of this chapter? If so, you may be able to *save as much as half* on your costs and copayments by asking your pharmacist if a tablet-splitting dose can save you money.

Many drugs cost the same regardless of tablet size. For example, a 20 mg Lipitor tablet costs almost exactly the same as the 40 mg version (and the 80 mg tablet, as well). So if you now take one 20 mg tablet per day, you can save up to $600 per year by asking your doctor to prescribe half a 40 mg tablet daily instead.

Many tablets are already scored across the middle by the manufacturer, and you simply break them in two with your hands. If not, you can buy an inexpensive tablet-splitter from any pharmacy. It's a small guillotine-like device that makes it easy to split tablets in two.

For years, doctors have found pill splitting to be a

safe practice for many of their patients. However, not every medication is appropriate for tablet splitting. For example, capsules, non-oral medications, extended release drugs, tablets with enteric coatings, tablets that crumble, tablets with nonsymmetric shapes, and drugs requiring precise dosages fall into this category. Also, not all patients are physically or mentally capable of using this method.

Tablet splitting is *not* something you should do without talking to your pharmacist or doctor—or both. A pharmacist can tell you if a drug is appropriate for splitting (and she's usually much easier to get on the telephone than your doctor). More importantly, your pharmacist actually knows how much each medication costs, so can tell you definitively if tablet splitting can save you money. Doctors often will not know enough about a drug's price to tell you if you can save money with this technique. But, of course, it is your doctor who must actually prescribe it before the pharmacist can dispense the drugs.

Here are some good rules of thumb to follow to find out if tablet splitting is right for you and your family:

Take inventory

Take out all of your family's regular medications and find out if any are on this chapter's list of drugs. They may be appropriate for tablet splitting. Note that I say *may be appropriate,* because not all tablet sizes are splittable, and sometimes even where tablet splitting is physically possible, it may not save you any money—it might even cost you more. That's why the following rules are also important.

Call or visit your pharmacist

Ask to speak with your pharmacist. Tell him which medications you are taking from the list and in what form and dosages, and ask whether you can save money by obtaining table-split doses instead of the formulation you now have. He can tell you if the double-strength tablets are splittable and how much you can save.

Ask your pharmacist to request new prescriptions

Once you find out that tablet splitting is appropriate, ask your pharmacist to call your doctor to request a new prescription. Most pharmacists will be happy to do this, but if not, just jot down the information and call your doctor yourself. Or better yet, go to another pharmacy. If you make the call to the doctor, you will most likely speak with the nurse who will forward your request to the doctor, and who, if it is approved, will call the new prescriptions in to your pharmacy.

New prescriptions

When your doctor writes a new prescription with you in her office, ask about tablet splitting then (Question #5). Doctors can usually quickly determine whether tablet splitting is physically feasible, but they will likely not know whether you will save money. Since most tablet-splitting prescriptions will save you money, go ahead and ask your doctor for it, and ask for a paper prescription rather than having the doctor phone it in to the pharmacy.

Talk to your pharmacist

When you already have a tablet-splitting prescription, take it to your pharmacy and ask to speak to the pharmacist. Ask him whether this prescription will save you money and how much. If you like the answer, then tell the pharmacist you want the prescription filled. If not, ask the pharmacist to call your doctor to change the prescription back to a lower cost version. This may sound like a lot to put your pharmacist and doctor through, but they are much more willing to do it for a patient than for an insurance company, so make sure they know that you are the one who is concerned about cost.

Splitting the tablet

- **Who should do it?** Only people who are physically able should attempt to split tablets. Thus, anyone with dexterity problems, vision problems, cognitive limitations, or physical disabilities (such as severe arthritis or Parkinson's disease) should have someone else do the tablet splitting.
- **Only when needed.** Once you split a tablet, the resulting pieces are much more likely to crumble if not taken immediately. Thus, you should only split the minimum number of tablets to meet your immediate needs. For this reason, you should not split a larger quantity, nor should you ask your pharmacist to split them for you.
- **Scored tablet.** If the manufacturer has already scored the tablet across the middle (or sometimes into thirds), you will find this is the easi-

est to split. Then it's a simple matter of pressing with your thumbs at the score and pulling against the ends of the pill with your forefingers. Voila! It's split. Scoring is also a pretty sure sign that the pill is appropriate for splitting. Still, if you have physical problems that prevent your doing this, you'll need help.

- **Tablet-splitter.** Virtually every drugstore and supermarket sells a guillotine-like pill-splitter for a few dollars. There are different designs, and some are better than others, depending on the size and shape of the pill you're splitting. However, the fact that they make and sell the things should give you confidence that pill splitting is an accepted, useful practice. Just place the tablet in the proper receptacle, lower the handle, and the cutting blade will split the pill.
- **Knife blade method.** Use a sharp knife, or a *single* edge razor blade, or a box cutter, or a . . . you get the idea. Just make sure the blade is sharp and spanking clean. Place the blade's edge on the midpoint of the pill, and press down until the pill splits. I have also successfully used a clean pair of sharp scissors. Some pills, like Glucophage (metformin), are especially hard, and can go flying when they finally do split. You can control this by covering the whole operation with a dry washcloth.

Tablet splitting has been used for years by doctors as a way to help their patients save money. There have been numerous articles supporting the practice in the medical literature.[1] Check it out to see if you can save money, too.

Potential Tablet-Split Drugs

(Note: brand name drugs are capitalized, generic drugs are lowercased.)

Accolate	Accupril	Aceon
Actos	acyclovir (Zovirax)	albuterol (Proventil)
allopurinol	alprazolam (Xanax)	Amaryl
Ambien	amitriptyline (Elavil)	amoxicillin (Amoxil)
amoxicillin/ clavulanate potassium (Augmentin)	Aricept	Atacand
atenolol (Tenormin)	Avandia	Avapro
Biaxin	buspirone (BuSpar)	Caduet
captopril (Capoten)	Celebrex	Celexa
cephalexin	clonazepam (Klonopin)	clonidine (Catapres)
Coreg	Coumadin	cyclobenzaprine (Flexeril)
diazepam (Valium)	diltiazem (Cardizem)	Diovan HCT
doxazosin (Cardura)	doxycycline	Effexor
enalapril	estropipate (Ortho-Est)	famotidine (Pepcid)
fluoxetine (Prozac)	furosemide (Lasix)	gemfibrozil (Lopid)

Potential Tablet-Split Drugs (cont'd)

(Note: brand name drugs are capitalized, generic drugs are lowercased.)

glipizide (Glucotrol)	glyburide (DiaBeta)	hydrochlorothiazide
hydrocodone with APAP (Vicodin)	hydroxyzine	ibuprofen (Advil)
isosorbide	labetalol (Normodyne)	Lanoxin
Levaquin	Levoxyl	Lipitor
lisinopril (Prinivil)	lorazepam (Ativan)	lovastatin (Mevacor)
meclizine (Bonine)	metformin (Glucophage)	methylprednisolone (Medrol)
metoclopramide (Reglan)	metoprolol (Toprol XL)	metronidazole
Monopril	Nadolol	naproxen (Naprosyn)
Norvasc	oxycodone with APAP (Percocet)	penicillin VK
Plavix	Pravachol	Premarin
promethazine (Phenergran)	propoxyphene with APAP (Darvocet)	propranolol (Inderal)
ranitidine (Zantac)	Risperdal (soon available as generic)	Seroquel

Potential Tablet-Split Drugs (cont'd)

(Note: brand name drugs are capitalized, generic drugs are lowercased.)

Singulair	Skelaxin	spironolactone (Aldactone)
Synthroid	Topamax	tramadol (Ultram)
trazodone	triamterene with HCTZ	trimethoprim with SMZ (Septra)
Univase	Valtrex	verapamil (Verelan)
Viagra	Zoloft	

CHAPTER 9

Free Samples, Free Lunch?

Several months ago, a Hyde Rx member called me to report her experience in asking her doctor the 7 Questions. She had visited her doctor for what turned out to be a chronic ear infection. After telling him that she had to pay a large percentage of her drug costs, she showed him the 7 Questions and asked him to help her save money on her prescription drug treatment. The doctor took a quick look at the questions and told her that he had previously prescribed generic antibiotics for her, and they had proved ineffective for her particular malady. She had acquired a bug that was resistant to the standard therapies. Unfortunately, he told her, she needed a new and very expensive brand name antibiotic. She then asked him again if there was anything he could do to help her save money; and he looked at the 7 Questions again, this time seeing Question #7 about extra free samples. He stood up, walked out of his office, and returned a few minutes later with a plastic shopping bag (with a brand name drug emblazoned on it) full of free samples of the antibiotic. He had actually given her the *entire course of treatment* of the antibiotic. She didn't have to pay for prescription drugs at all. After I congratulated her on her savvy behavior, she asked me how much her free drugs were worth. I looked it up on my computer and found that her doctor had given her $290 worth of drugs!

Another member told me that she gets weekly allergy shots at her doctor's office and that she asks for free samples of her brand name antihistamine medication every time. She said that during the past year, she received almost all the drugs she needed this way—absolutely free.

I hear stories like this a lot.

Every year drug manufacturers practically beg doctors to accept shovels full of samples of expensive brand name medications to give to their patients. The retail value of these free drugs amounts to hundreds of millions of dollars per year. Lest you think this is out of some charitable impulse, let me hasten to add that the drug companies know that if they can get a patient started on an immediately available, free medication, they are much more likely to continue to use that drug for the duration of their condition. And the duration of many chronic conditions is a lifetime. A single chronic-disease patient represents a future potential revenue stream to the drug companies of many thousands of dollars.

There are now so many drug reps trying to get face time that doctors are increasingly limiting or even refusing access to them. One method that sales reps use to get in is to require a doctor to personally sign a receipt for his free sample deliveries. Since a single delivery can amount to thousands of dollars worth of drugs, most doctors want them, and are willing to spend a few brief minutes with the rep in order to get them.

Nonetheless, there is an increasing trend toward doctors refusing both to see the drug reps and to accept free samples. Some physician medical groups are even setting up their own pharmacy and therapeutics committees (P&T committees) to independently evaluate and recommend drugs to their colleagues in the group, rather than relying on the heavily biased drug reps for their information.

Despite the high cost of sampled drugs, there are times when free samples can be a good thing for patients like the two Hyde Rx members mentioned above. For one thing, patients are more likely to start taking needed medications earlier than they would if they had to wait to get a prescription filled. This is particularly helpful for acute ailments, such as infections. And for patients who might just let a paper prescription sit on their counter for months without getting it filled, it provides an extra nudge to get started on potentially life-enhancing drugs.

For patients without insurance coverage, these free drugs from a sympathetic doctor can sometimes supply all their prescription needs at no cost. Obviously, the drug companies don't intend for this to be too widespread a practice, but they are aware it happens and tolerate it as a necessary cost of doing business. Besides, they can always point this out as a positive aspect of their own munificence and desire to make drugs more affordable.

So, if there are all these free drugs available for the asking, why didn't I just say this at the beginning of the book instead of making you wait until Chapter 9? Isn't free good? No, it may not be. Remember the old saying, "There's no such thing as a free lunch." I have written elsewhere in this book about the tendency of doctors to unintentionally saddle their patients with high drug costs by giving them a handful of free samples and a prescription for the same stuff. Prices on such drugs are much higher than for generics and other alternatives. What is the benefit of your doctor starting you on a two-week free sample of a brand name medication that will end up costing you $90 per month when the sample runs out, when instead he could have prescribed a therapeutically equivalent generic drug costing only $10?

This raises an obvious question; why not just ask the doctor for free generic drug samples instead of brand name ones? Unfortunately, unlike the brand name drug manufacturers, generic drug makers almost never give free samples to doctors. Once a brand name drug loses its patent protection, it becomes a public domain commodity that can be made by any number of competing companies. Since the FDA assures that all generics are chemically and therapeutically equivalent to the original brand name, there is no way for a given manufacturer to differentiate its particular version on the basis of quality, safety, or effectiveness—they are all the same. That leaves price as the primary mode for competing. A given pharmacy might stock a drug from Company R this week and then switch to Company S's version next week, because the price is better. Thus, there is no point in a generic drug company giving away free samples, since there's no way for that company to assure that the patient will actually end up buying its drugs at the pharmacy.

Sometimes doctors may receive free generic drug samples from HMOs or health insurance companies they do business with. This is not a widespread practice, however, so unless you live in California or one of the other handful of states with such programs, you're out of luck.

For the vast majority of patients, if you want generics, you'll just have to pay for them. The good news, of course, is that you will normally see huge savings from foregoing the enticing "free lunch" drug samples and then paying for a lifetime of the stuff. So when your doctor offers you free samples, tell her that you have to pay for your own drugs and want an equivalent generic drug if available. If you happen to know the retail price of the sample medication, tell your doctor. Surprisingly few physicians know how much these drugs actually cost. Giving her this information can help sensitize her to this issue for her other patients and start her thinking more about generics as a first line of medication defense.

But let's say that, for your particular condition, a generic medication has proved ineffective or is simply unavailable. In that case, a brand name drug may be your only option. If that's the case, then free samples can save you a lot of money. Again, explain to your doctor that you have limited or no insurance coverage and must pay for your own drugs, and would he please load you up with free samples. Try to get enough to tide you over until your next visit when you can renew your supply. Or your doctor may ask you to drop by every few weeks for more, so that he doesn't suddenly deplete his inventory in supplying you.

But also take another look at the "Drug Classes by Cost" table in Chapter 7 and notice that some brand name drugs within a therapeutic class are considerably less expensive than others. Armed with this information before your doctor visit, you can ask if a less expensive one may be appropriate for you. Then if you are not able to get sufficient samples, at least you'll be paying less for your treatment.

Here are some simple rules for making sure you always get the maximum number of free samples:

1. **Last resort.** Remember that free samples are preferable only if there are no effective alternatives to such expensive brand name drugs.

2. **Don't be shy.** Always remember that your doctor gets his sample supply for free, and that there are more where those came from. Don't be embarrassed about asking for extra when he hands you a starter supply with a prescription for more. Just explain that you need to pay for your drugs, and ask politely.

3. **Come back for more.** If you ask for extras and are told that they are running low, ask if you can call them in a week or two to see if they have been replenished. Also, whenever you or a family member visits your doctor for any reason, always ask if you can please have more samples.

4. **Don't forget tablet splitting.** While you're at it, ask your doctor to give you double-dose sample tablets if he has them and if they can be split. These can double your supply.

Free samples can be a problematical way to get drugs if they prevent you from buying less expensive generics or OTC meds that would work just as well for you. But if there are no such options, free samples can be a useful way to stretch your healthcare dollars.

CHAPTER 10

Free and Discounted Drug Programs

Once you have your prescription, there are many ways you can save money when you actually purchase your drugs. Even if you have good health insurance, don't ignore this chapter, as you may find a few surprises that can help you save. If you are one of the millions of Americans with limited or no prescription drug insurance coverage, this chapter can save you hundreds or thousands of dollars a year in out-of-pocket drug costs. At any given time, there are about 45 million people with no health insurance at all, and many millions more who have limited or no coverage for prescription drugs. (I personally fall into this category, since I have a high deductible health insurance policy that has no drug coverage at all.)

Regardless of our income or insurance coverage, though, none of us want to pay more than we have to for *anything*, especially prescription drugs. For many of us, saving money on prescription drugs is a simple matter of thrift. But for the more than 29 million people who have low income and are uninsured, this chapter could mean the difference between getting their drugs and doing without.

This chapter will tell you how to minimize your drug costs by using the following programs and techniques (Note: Medicare's new drug benefit is covered in Chapter 13):

Medicaid

Veterans benefits

Patient assistance
programs

Commercial discount
memberships and
cards

Community health
centers

Rebates and coupons

Drug trials

MEDICAID

Almost 15 million[1] of America's 45 million uninsured are actually eligible for government assistance programs such as Medicaid, but have failed to apply. Medicaid is a government-sponsored entitlement program that pays for medical services and prescription drugs for people with low incomes and limited resources, especially children, pregnant women, and the disabled. A joint federal and state system, Medicaid now covers 53 million people and includes 25 million children. It costs $300 billion a year—more than Medicare.[2]

It is not always easy to figure out if you are eligible for Medicaid, but if you are, you will find their prescription drug coverage, which varies from state-to-state, to be generally excellent. Just be aware that any program that produces a "Brief Summary" of itself that runs to twelve single-spaced typewritten pages is not going to be especially easy to navigate.[3] Medicaid is, after all, a government program and one that has been continually tweaked, modified, limited, expanded, and amended for the forty-plus years it has been in existence. There is nothing simple about it.

Here is a brief summary that is considerably shorter than twelve pages:

If you (or your children) are temporarily or permanently poor or near poor, you may be able to receive medical and prescription drug benefits from your state's Medicaid program. There are more than twenty-five different patient eligibility categories that the federal government helps to fund. In general, these include low-income pregnant women; children and teenagers; and people who are aged, blind, and disabled. Here are some of the categories of people who are generally eligible, although the specifics vary widely from state to state:

- Those who meet the old AFDC (Aid to Families with Dependent Children) program requirements.

- Those under age six with family income less than 133% of the Federal Poverty Level (FPL).

- Those under age nineteen with family income less than the FPL.

- Pregnant women with family income below 135% of the FPL (services are limited to pregnancy-related conditions).

- SSI (Supplemental Security Income) recipients in most states.

- Recipients of adoption or foster care assistance under the Social Security Act.

- Special protected groups who may keep Medicaid even after losing eligibility for cash assistance programs.

- Some Medicare beneficiaries.

- Additional groups in some states, with looser criteria than required for the above.

I told you it's complicated. While prescription drugs are technically classified as optional services under Medicaid, most—if not all—states and territories provide such coverage, often at little or no cost to patients.

The best way to find out if you or your children are eligible for Medicaid is to call the U.S. government's Centers for Medicare and Medicaid Services toll-free at 877-267-2323. It's an automated, menu-driven, voice-activated response system that requires a little patience to navigate, but if you dial and say the right things, you will receive the telephone number for your state's Medicaid agency. Then call that number to find out if you are eligible and how to apply.

VETERANS BENEFITS

If you are a registered military veteran, you can get most of your VA doctor–prescribed prescriptions filled at nominal cost at a Department of Veterans Affairs hospital or outpatient clinic. For information, go to www.va.gov, call the VA toll-free at 877-222-8387, or contact your local Veterans' Agent Office or VA healthcare facility. At this writing, registered vets can obtain a 30-day supply for a $7 copayment, although there are rumblings about increasing the cost to $15. If your prescription is for generic drugs, you may actually find it cheaper to get it filled elsewhere and pay cash. (See Chapter 11 for details.)

PATIENT ASSISTANCE PROGRAMS

A couple of years ago, I received a call from a Hyde Rx member whose child suffered from a rare genetic disorder and required ongoing injections of genetically engineered medications at a total cost of several thousand dollars a month. The mother had limited income from her factory job, and despite partial insurance coverage, still found herself having to pay more than a thousand dollars a month for the drug, which she simply could not afford. After discussing the cost problem with the mother, I asked one of my colleagues to see if there was a free drug program that could help the mother and her child. We reported our findings to the mother who was able to apply for and receive complete forgiveness of her financial burden for the drugs. The child continued to receive her injections, and I recently learned that she is healthy, normal, and now completely off the medication.

Few people realize that drug manufacturers offer more than 150 free drug programs under which low-income patients can receive their needed drugs for free. In addition, there are at least 125 similar programs operated by state and local governments and by charitable organizations that also offer free drugs for low-income individuals. And there are many more additional discount programs offered by drug companies for people who are not eligible for free drugs, but who can still save considerable sums on their medications. An estimated two billion dollars' worth of free medications are given away annually, but there has been very little publicity about them. As a result, many otherwise eligible patients are either spending more than they need to or, worse, going without much-needed medications.

So, the good news is that there are currently more than 275 patient assistance programs that offer more than 1,200 drugs on a no-cost or low-cost basis to qualifying patients. The bad news is that there are more than 275 patient assistance programs for you to attempt to wade through in order to find one or more that can work for you.

Fortunately, there is now a single free access point for almost all of these programs. It is called the Partnership for Prescription Assistance (PPA). PPA is a nonprofit partnership of drug companies, healthcare providers, patient advocates, and community groups that provides assistance to uninsured and low-income patients who may have difficulty paying for their medications. Through it, you can quickly—and at no charge—determine which programs are the most likely to offer what you need.

Each of these 275 or so programs has its own set of requirements for eligibility. However, most are aimed at patients who have no prescription drug coverage and whose personal income falls below 200% of the Federal Poverty Level—this works out to about $19,000 for an individual and $31,000 for a family of three. PPA estimates that more than 29 million people in the United States make less than 200% of the federal poverty level and are uninsured.[4] If these criteria apply to you, or to a relative, friend, or neighbor, then check it out.

Other PPA programs are available to anyone who lacks prescription drug insurance coverage—regardless of income level. Just remember that actual qualifications vary from program to program and even from state to state, so you should not assume that you don't qualify just because you don't fit the above financial criteria. There may still be a program that fits your needs.

Identifying which of these programs may be appropriate for you is relatively easy. You can call PPA toll-free at 1-888-477-2669, although the process is much faster and easier if you just go to their website at www.pparx.org. I am a big proponent of consumers using the Internet to help find the drugs they need at the lowest possible price. This website is a good example of a powerful, if somewhat quirky, online resource that can quickly direct drug consumers to potentially hundreds or even thousands of dollars in annual savings.

Whether you call or go to the website (once on their homepage, select "Patients Click Here to Start"). You will be asked by the operator or website to select all the drugs that you currently are taking. Once you've done that, you will then be asked:

- Your age
- State of residence
- Zip code
- Yearly household income
- How many people in your household
- Whether you are pregnant

- Your current residency status
  - ❏ U.S. citizen
  - ❏ Legal resident of the U.S.
  - ❏ Other
- Whether you are eligible for any of the following (note that most drug assistance programs will disqualify you if you participate in any of these programs, although prescription drug discount cards are usually OK):
  - ❏ Medicare
  - ❏ Medicaid
  - ❏ Veteran's assistance
  - ❏ HMO/PPO
  - ❏ State insurance
  - ❏ Private insurance
  - ❏ Prescription drug coverage for the medicines entered previously
  - ❏ None
  - ❏ Do not know
- How did you hear about pparx.org? (You can answer "Friend." We are friends, right?)

After entering this information, the site or operator will tell you about your eligibility for one or more of these programs. Please note that some are for free drugs and others for discounts. You can then ask about or click on each program to learn the details about the organization offering it, and then decide if you wish to apply.

Once you've found the appropriate program or

programs online, there are usually two different ways to apply. One is to click on the particular program on the website and download an application form (or call to have it sent to you). You must then print, complete, and submit the application along with the supporting financial and other documentation required by each program. Please note that each program has its own application form. Thus, if you are taking drugs made by three different companies, you'll need to complete and submit three different applications—a time-consuming task.

The second, and easiest, way is to use the online Application Wizard to fill out multiple applications at once. If you are applying for more than one program, the Application Wizard is much easier than filling out forms by hand, although I found it somewhat challenging to use. Some questions and instructions are unclear, and I hope these usability problems will be addressed by the time you read these words.

As you complete the application, you will find that you may be required to provide some very personal, private information such as your Social Security Number, your race, and details about your financial condition. Many programs (especially the ones for free drugs) also require proof of financial condition, such as copies of your income tax returns. You will also need to get your doctor to complete part of any application for free drugs from manufacturers.

Once you've completed the Application Wizard, the website will then complete each application, which you must then individually print. You will still need to review each one, proofread it, sign it, provide any required supporting documentation, and mail it to the proper address. In testing the initial version of the Application Wizard, I found a number of gaps in the information actually transferred to the applications, so you'll need to proofread and correct each one before submitting it.

The actual programs differ widely as to where they actually deliver your medications (i.e., to you or to your doctor) and how long your initial application is good for (e.g., a single 90-day fill or multiple fills).

All of the participating programs in Partnership for Prescription Assistance claim to provide strong privacy protection, but not all may be subject to the legal protection of the federal Health Insurance Portability and Accountability Act (HIPAA). Even if you utilize the PPA website for completing your application(s), you may wish to telephone each program for privacy assurances before actually mailing the application.

In addition to PPA, AARP also operates a website with a state-by-state listing of patient assistance programs, although it is not as comprehensive as the PPA site. You can find it at http://www.aarp.org/bulletin/prescription/Articles/statebystate.html.

One final note. On the Internet, you can find a number of so-called free-drug websites that charge you for the same information you can get for free from www.pparx.org or from the individual sponsor websites. You don't need to pay for this information.

COMMERCIAL DISCOUNT MEMBERSHIPS AND CARDS

If you don't qualify for one of the above needs-based patient assistance programs, you may still be able to

benefit from one of a multitude of drug discount cards
and memberships that are available through a variety
of companies, employers, and associations. Like patient assistance programs, these discount programs
are not insurance. Unlike patient assistance programs,
they usually have the following characteristics:

- No eligibility requirements. Anyone can sign up.
- A one-time or annual enrollment fee and/or a
  per-prescription charge (often included in the
  total drug cost).
- Discounts available from participating retail
  pharmacies.
- Mail order pharmacy fulfillment, often with
  lower prices and greater quantities than available at retail (some programs offer only mail
  order discounts).

Here's how they work. The sponsors of the discount cards negotiate discounts directly with pharmacies, sometimes many thousands of pharmacies. In
addition, they may negotiate a rebate arrangement
from the pharmacies for each prescription and from
drug manufacturers for specific brand name drugs.
Thus, the sponsor may receive substantial undisclosed
revenue in addition to the membership fees.

It is important to understand that the discounts
with such card programs are not calculated on a pharmacy's retail price of the drug. Instead, discounts are
usually applied to the drug's average wholesale price,
or AWP. This is not a number you'll likely be able to
find anywhere. In fact AWP is increasingly viewed as a
convenient fiction by which drug manufacturers, dis-

tributors, and retailers are able to maintain artificially high prices for drugs. Some observers say that AWP actually stands for "ain't what's paid." This is doubly true for generic drugs, in which the AWP is often many times the price you can get at retail. In short, even a big AWP discount, such as 40–50%, can still yield a higher price than you might otherwise pay after doing a little comparison shopping.

Even though discount card programs are not insurance, they may impose insurance-like limits on the amount of drugs you can receive with each prescription, especially for retail pharmacy purchases. There are at least three reasons for this. First, by limiting you to a 30-day supply of drugs with each retail purchase of your maintenance medications, the sponsor may receive more in prescription-based rebates from the fulfilling pharmacy than if they allowed you to purchase 90-day supplies. Second, the pharmacy, which charges you a dispensing fee each time a prescription is filled, will get to charge it more frequently on your maintenance medications than if you were allowed to purchase greater quantities. Pharmacies usually include the dispensing fee in the total drug price, so you may not be aware that it is being charged. Third, by limiting you to 30-days at retail, but 90-days at mail order, the plan sponsor can divert you to its own highly profitable mail order pharmacy operation.

Recently, a member of my family ran out of a maintenance medication and needed it refilled immediately at a retail pharmacy. I had learned from previous comparison shopping experiences (see Chapter 11) that a national discount club store across town usually offered the lowest prices locally, so I took the prescription there. When I presented the 90-day quantity prescription at the pharmacy window, I asked two questions:

1. How much will it cost with my prescription drug discount card? (I don't have drug insurance.)
2. How much would it cost without the discount card at your full retail price?

It turned out that the discount card offered a slight savings over the retail price, so I asked the pharmacy clerk to use the card. But when I returned to get the drugs, I discovered that the pharmacist had dispensed only a 30-day supply rather than the 90-day supply indicated on the prescription. When I pointed this out, I was told that the discount card company had indicated on the pharmacy's computer screen that only a 30-day supply was allowed, so that's all they filled.

Rather than accept this, I again confirmed how much a 90-day supply of the same drug would cost without the discount card. The answer was that the full retail cash price for 90-days was less than three times the discounted cost of the 30-day supply. In other words, if I paid full retail for a 90-day supply *without* the discount card, I would pay less per tablet than if I purchased a 30-day supply *with* the discount card. I decided to forget the discount card and go for the higher quantity and lower cost. It is likely that the lower price resulted from the fact that I was paying the same dispensing fee for the 90-day supply as I would have for the 30-day supply.

I have learned from this and other experiences that discount card prices are not always cheaper than full retail, especially when you include the annual membership fee. It is important to always comparison shop among different pharmacies to find the best price, with or without a discount card.

By the way, when I have called pharmacies to ask about drug prices with my discount card, they have rarely given me prices over the phone. But when asked for their full retail "cash price," they always give it to me. To find the discount card price, I have to call the discount card sponsor's phone number on the card. If I don't have time to call, I always take the prescription to the lowest cash price pharmacy and do my comparison pricing there. As often as not, I end up paying the cash price, especially when I want a 90-day supply, but that's probably because I have access to a warehouse club pharmacy. If you only have access to regular independent or chain drugstores, a discount card may make a lot more sense for you.

So never assume that a discount card will save you more money than comparison shopping alone (again see Chapter 11), especially if you have the option of waiting for mail order delivery. Before buying such a card, do your homework to see if you can get your drugs cheaper without it. Call the company and ask them exactly how much your own prescriptions will cost, and whether their discounts are available at your particular local pharmacies. Then call the pharmacies for their cash prices. You may find you don't need the card.

There are many sources for obtaining discount cards. A relatively easy way to check out your options is to enter "prescription drug discount card" or a similar phrase in your computer's Internet search engine (e.g., Google, Teoma, Yahoo). You'll find there are many, many such programs being offered. Another approach is to ask your local pharmacy if they offer a discount program. You will find a wide variety of discount cards ranging from those that are good at a single pharmacy chain to those you can use at more than

50,000 pharmacies. Promised discounts range from 40% to 80%. Membership fees range from free to $15 a month—or more.

In evaluating your discount card options, I recommend the following:

DO:

1. Do identify several competing discount card programs through an Internet search engine, advertisements, and by calling local pharmacies.
2. Do check to see if they have participating pharmacies near where you live or work.
3. Do create a list of all the drugs you and your family are now taking, along with how much you are currently paying for them and how much you spend per year. (Appendix B provides a worksheet for this purpose.)
4. Do calculate the annual cost of your drugs under each discount card plan. Don't forget to include any membership fees for the card itself, taking into account whether each program covers your entire family or only a single individual.
5. Do check your results by going to my website at www.HydeRx.com to compare the results of your analysis with the prices from Hyde Rx's linked pharmacies.
6. Do check out the business reputation of your preferred programs. Contact your state attorney general's office or Better Business Bureau for a history of unresolved complaints.
7. Do sign up for the program that gives you the lowest total cost over a year's time. You may

find it advantageous to sign up for more than one program.

8. Before renewing an existing discount card, do try to find a better one. Be particularly wary of any program that starts you off with low prices, but then increases them during the year—particularly for generic drugs.

DON'T:

1. Don't click on or sign up for *any* discount drug scheme offered to you by unsolicited spam e-mail. You're asking for trouble if you do.

2. Don't sign up for any program that won't tell you the prices of your specific drugs, either over the Internet or by telephone.

3. Don't pay a lot of attention to claims of high percentage discounts. Most apply only to generic drug prices that you may be able to beat with comparison shopping without any discount card. Brand name drug discounts will be far lower than the maximums quoted. In any event, you don't care about the amount of the discount. You care about getting the lowest price.

Grocery Chain Loyalty Program Discounts

A number of grocery chains are now offering discounts on drugs to their uninsured customers who show a store loyalty card.[5] Since the cards are free and offer discount savings on many other store items, you probably already have one or more of the cards. I have three. Discounts on generics can be as high as 60%. Be sure to ask your grocery store pharmacies if they offer such discounts. Just make sure you also do your comparison shopping (Chapter 11).

COMMUNITY HEALTH CENTERS

The Community Health Centers program of the U.S. Public Health Service provides grants to more than 700 community-based nonprofit organizations that operate more than 3,000 health clinics in rural and medically underserved areas across the United States.[6] These clinics provide a wide range of low-cost health-care services, including prescription drugs, primary and preventive care, lab tests, X-rays health education, and more to the residents of their communities. These CHC clinics serve more than 11 million people.

Community Health Centers and their federally qualified look-alike brethren are able to participate in the government's 340B Drug Pricing Program. This allows them to purchase prescription drugs at much deeper discounts than are available for commercial pharmacies. These facilities then offer these drugs to their patients at low cost. If you have access to such a facility, give them a call to find out if they can save you money on your prescription drugs. While you may find their prices to be attractive, they may also require that all prescriptions be written by their own doctors. Be sure to ask.

To find the nearest CHC, go to the website at http://ask.hrsa.gov/pc/ and enter your location. There does not appear to be a telephone number for those who are unable to access this website. The website search function does not let you specify pharmacy services as a search criterion, but you can call any centers that you do find to ask whether they have a pharmacy, how you can utilize it, and how much they charge for their drugs. The savings can be significant.

REBATES AND COUPONS

Some drug companies offer money-back coupons, rebates, or free samples if you buy their brand name drugs. I'm not a big fan of these programs, since they encourage people to buy drugs that are more expensive than other lower cost, equally effective drugs. However, if you have done your homework and consulted your doctor and pharmacist about the 7 Questions and find that one of these drugs is really best for you, then these programs can help you save some money.

On the following pages, I've listed some of the programs that are available as of this writing. If you don't see your drugs listed here, most brand name drugs have their own dedicated websites where you can check to see if there are any money-saving offers. These programs are subject to change at any time, and of course, you'll still have to get a doctor's prescription for each drug. You can find most of these websites by just entering www.*drugname*.com, where you type in the actual drug name for *drugname*. If that doesn't work, then type the drug name into one of the Internet search engines (e.g., www.google.com, www.teoma.com, or www.yahoo.com) to find the official site.

Rebate/Free Sample/Coupon Programs

Drug	Treats	Offer	Website	Telephone
AcipHex	Acid reflux	Up to $30 refund	www.aciphex.com	800-526-7736
Allegra	Allergies	Up to $140 rebate	www.allegra.com	800-262-2827
Cialis	Erectile dysfunction	2 free samples	www.cialis.com	877-242-5471
Clarinex	Allergies	$10 rebate	www.clarinex.com	
Comtan	Parkinson's disease	30-day free supply	www.comtan.com	888-669-6682
Elidel	Eczema	$10 off	www.elidel.com	888-669-6682
Exelon	Alzheimer's disease	30-day free supply	www.exelon.com	888-669-6682
Famvir	Genital herpes	5-day or 2-week free supply	www.genitalherpes.com	888-669-6682

Rebate/Free Sample/Coupon Programs (cont'd)

Drug	Treats	Offer	Website	Telephone
Lamisil	Toenail fungus	$10 off or 7-day supply	www.lamisil.com	888-669-6682
Levitra	Erectile dysfunction	Buy 1, get 1 free, up to 8 tablets (requires you to divulge personal information & permit advertising be sent to you)	www.levitra.com	888-825-5249
Nexium	Acid reflux	7-day free supply	www.purplepill.com	800-236-9933
Ortho Evra	Birth control	$5 off	www.orthoevra.com	800-682-6532
Prevacid	Acid reflux	7-day free supply	www.prevacid.com	800-621-1020
Protonix	Acid reflux	$30 refund	www.protonix.com	
Zelnorm	Chronic constipation	$10 off or 5-day free supply	www.zelnorm.com	888-669-6682
Zyrtec	Allergies	$20 refund	www.zyrtec.com	

DRUG TRIALS

One potential way to get free drugs is to become a human volunteer for a clinical drug trial. At any given time, there are hundreds of such studies being conducted by researchers from drug companies, governmental institutions, universities, and private foundations. Depending on the trial and what's being tested, qualified patients may be given a standard treatment drug, an experimental drug, a placebo, or no treatment at all.

While any drugs administered to you during a clinical trial will be entirely free, you will have no say in what drug, if any, you will actually get. You won't even know what you're getting when you get it. A key element of such *double-blind studies* is that neither the patient nor the doctor actually knows what's in the pill you are being asked to consume. And even if you happen to receive a medication that helps your condition, it is unlikely that you will continue to receive it once the trial is completed. Clinical trials are designed for the needs of the researcher, not the patient, so should not be viewed as a first-line option for finding affordable drugs.

The best way to find a trial that may work for you is to go to http://www.clinicaltrials.gov/, where you can search an extensive database of programs for which volunteers are being sought. The site provides an interactive search box into which you can enter one or more key words (e.g., "heart attack, Los Angeles"), and you will be able to browse all the various registered programs that fit your criteria. Just click on any program that looks interesting. I warn you that the language tends to be technical, but you may find something that looks interesting. If you do, you can contact the program via the contact information provided in the project description.

CONCLUSION

Many people are missing out on thousands of dollars worth of free drugs or discounted drugs through the programs described here. Find out if you're one of them.

CHAPTER 11

Savvy Shopping: Getting the Best Deal from Retail, Mail Order, and Internet Pharmacies

A while back, a newspaper reported that Arizona and Michigan have opened a new front in the states' war on prescription-drug prices. Arizona's then attorney general (now governor) Janet Napolitano was shocked (shocked!) to find that different pharmacies charge different prices for identical drugs. Likewise, Michigan's then AG Jennifer Granholm (also now governor) discovered that the arthritis medication Celebrex cost $78.98 at one Flint pharmacy and $96.22 at another. Ms. Granholm said she would bring price-gouging charges against any store her office concluded was overcharging. Ms. Napolitano was more reserved in her threats, saying ominously, "I want to get my facts first, before we decide what to do with all this information."[1]

I suppose many would applaud Ms. Napolitano and Ms. Granholm for bringing such seemingly rapacious behavior to light. Isn't it somehow unseemly that two different pharmacies are charging different prices for the same drug? After all, you might argue, prescription drugs are an essential part of a productive, functional life, and all drugs should be available to patients at the lowest cost, right? If such abuses are allowed to get out of hand, where might it end? What other essential products and services could succumb to the heartbreak of variable pricing? Next on this slippery slope we could even find supermarkets trying to charge different prices for an even more essential commodity—food. Wouldn't we risk having people starving in the streets if we allowed Safeway to charge more than Ralph's.

Of course we all know that supermarkets do compete on price, and very aggressively at that. So do stockbrokers, appliance stores, clothiers, and car dealers. Instead of hyperventilating about differential drug pricing, I prefer to take advantage of the opportunity created by the drugstores out there charging *less* than others for prescription drugs. I'm obviously not running for governor. Savvy Rx shoppers have a major opportunity to save a lot of money by shopping around.

A while back, I came down with a nasty respiratory infection, probably from sitting on too many airplanes. My doctor prescribed a generic drug (of course) to relieve my symptoms, and while I was waiting to get my chest x-rayed; I borrowed a telephone book and wrote down the numbers of three different pharmacies that my family uses. I called all three from my cell phone to see which one offered the lowest price for my script.

Even I was surprised by the range of prices on this common generic. A nationwide discount chain store pharmacy quoted $16. My friendly neighborhood supermarket pharmacist quoted $42. (So that's why he's so friendly!) But the Sam's Club pharmacy was the one that truly shocked me: $6 for the same drug, same number of doses. You don't have to guess what I did, even though Sam's was clear across town. I'm always willing to burn a little extra gas to save $36.

This is not an unusual experience, especially for generic drugs. Many drugstores mark up their generic prices many times above their low wholesale costs. Even after steep markups, they are still cheaper than most brand name drugs.

I now keep the phone numbers of several pharmacies in my pocket organizer for those occasions when I need to get a medication quickly. Otherwise, I just go home and look up the drug on the Internet to find a low mail order price. This works really well when I don't need the medication filled immediately, since there are several mail order pharmacies that always seem to offer the lowest prices for anyone who can afford to wait a few days.

For people without prescription drug insurance—or those with insurance who have to pay high out-of-pocket amounts—buying drugs shouldn't be any different than finding the lowest price for food, clothing, or cars; drugs are another essential, life-enhancing consumer item to be purchased at the lowest available price.

The problem is that it's easier to find the price for celery than it is for Celebrex. Because most drug customers have insurance, actual drug prices don't matter that much to them. As a result, pharmacies don't advertise their drug prices on TV or in your local paper, and you never see big sales promotions. Rx prices aren't even posted in the vast majority of pharmacies (or their websites), even though every other item in the store has a prominently displayed price tag.

I recently read an article about how the giant General Motors Corporation was paying a supposedly discounted price for three-month prescriptions of generic Zantac of $181.22 each, even though Wal-Mart was selling the same drug for $78.62, and Costco had it priced for $22.00![2] Moreover, the Wal-Mart and Costco prices were their full retail cash prices with no insurance discounts. If that story doesn't convince you of the value of shopping around for the best drug price, then I despair.

Unfortunately, many self-pay consumers don't know how much a drug will cost them until they pick it up at the pharmacy window, and even then, they aren't aware that they may have been able to get the same drug for 20–80% less at a nearby pharmacy. Generic drugs get the biggest markups at many pharmacies, and provide the greatest opportunity for savings, although brand name drug prices very widely as well. For example, a Texas consumer with a prescription for a generic version of Cipro antibiotic recently found the following prices at three different pharmacies:[3]

$84.59   Major chain pharmacy
$36.00   Canadian Internet pharmacy
$10.22   Local pharmacy

That's right; the independently owned local pharmacy offered a savings of more than 85% over the nationwide chain and more than 70% over the Canadian pharmacy.

Likewise, a Sacramento, California, consumer found that ninety tablets of brand name Lipitor were priced at $321.95 at a local regional chain store and at $193.77 at a nearby national club store pharmacy—a savings of 40% for this hugely popular cholesterol drug.[4]

These savings opportunities are not well known. Less than 10% of drug buyers actually engage in comparison shopping.[5] Not that it's all that easy. You may have to dig a bit, but it's worth the dig. A few minutes on the phone or Internet can yield big savings. Here's how to go about it.

STEP 1: TAKE INVENTORY

Get out all your family's current medications and prescriptions and create a spreadsheet like the one on the following page.

You can do it on paper or on your computer. Regardless of how you do it, the point is to write down in one place all the drugs that you and your next of kin take on a regular basis. List all drugs by family member. Under "Drug Name, Form, & Dose" you would write, for example, Allegra 180 mg tablets. Under "Drug Purpose" write the condition it treats, such as allergies, depression, high blood pressure, pain, etc. Below, I'll tell you how to determine quantities and prices for the rest of the spreadsheet.

STEP 2: DETERMINE QUANTITY LIMITATIONS

As with laundry detergent, the larger the quantity of drugs that you can buy at one time, the lower the price you will usually pay on a per-dose basis. Not only can you save money with quantity discounts, but you can also save on dispensing fees. Most retail pharmacies add a dispensing fee of two or three dollars for each prescription they fill. This fee is in addition to the price

Medication Spreadsheet

Family Mbr	Drug Name, Dose, & Form	Refill Date	Drug Purpose	Store Name 1:		Store Name 2:		Store Name 3:		Store Name 4:	
				Quant	Price	Quant	Price	Quant	Price	Quant	Price

of the drug product. Thus, if you're buying a 100-day supply, you should pay the same dispensing fee that you would for a 30-day supply, so your cost per pill goes down. If you are taking several medications, the amount you save in a year's time can be meaningful.

Also, you can often get a better deal on 100-pill quantities than on the more commonly prescribed 30-day or 90-day supplies. Many pharmacies receive their drugs packaged in manufacturer-sealed 100-tablet bottles. If you can order in multiples of that quantity, the pharmacist doesn't have to open any bottles and count out the pills, but instead can just stick a new label on the factory-sealed packages. This can result in a lower price, and it also reduces the risk of pharmacist error.

Another advantage of buying in larger quantities is that you get to skip interim price increases in the drug. Many brand name drug manufacturers increase their prices several times a year. In 2004, brand prices increased by 7.1%[6] (the general inflation rate was only 2.6%), and in April 2005 alone, prescription drug prices rose[7] at an annualized rate of 11.4%! If you can buy a three month's, six month's, or even a year's supply of your drugs at today's lower price, you'll spend less than if you get your drugs a month at a time.

There are two potential downsides to quantity orders. First, your upfront outlay will be significantly higher than when you buy only a 30-day supply. Of course, you save money over the longer term, but it can be a problem if cash is tight. Second, if you subsequently discover that the drug doesn't work for you or causes unwanted side effects, you could end up with a bunch of useless pills. Pharmacies do not accept returns. Make sure any drug works for you before committing to large quantities.

If you have insurance or use a drug discount card,

the pharmacy benefit manager (PBM) will almost always limit the quantities you can buy. Most PBMs will limit you to a 30-day supply for retail prescriptions and a 90-day supply for mail order. They do this in order to drive as many patients as possible to their own highly profitable mail service operations. And they do not allow their members to use any other mail service pharmacy—only their own.

If you don't know what your quantity limits are, you can easily find out. Call the phone number on your drug ID card and ask what kind of quantity limitations the company imposes on retail and mail order prescriptions for maintenance drugs. Ask specifically if they allow 90-day or 100-day limits at retail. Also ask if you can get 100-day supplies from mail order.

If you have no drug insurance or discount card, then there won't be any such artificial limits on the quantities of drugs you can buy at retail or mail, except for narcotics and other controlled substances that are usually quantity-limited by state law. Otherwise, the only limitations will be those imposed by your doctor, generally for reasons of safety or efficacy. In general, you will find it to your long-term financial advantage to buy in the largest practical quantities, such as 100-day supplies or more.

Once you've determined your quantity limits, enter them for each drug in your drug inventory spreadsheet.

STEP 3: COMPARE PRICES

The next step is to conduct some plain old comparison shopping. Pull out your telephone directory, and look up several local pharmacies. Try to include at least one independent pharmacy, a chain pharmacy, and a club store pharmacy (e.g., Sam's or Costco). If you have a grocery store loyalty program that offers discounted drug costs, be sure to include it. Keep these phone numbers in any address book or PDA that you carry with you. Then enter the pharmacy names and contact information in your spreadsheet. If you have insurance or a drug discount card, always make sure these pharmacies are in your approved network.

Be sure to add mail service pharmacies to your list. They often cost less than retail, although the main drawback to mail service is that you have to wait a couple of days to a couple of weeks for delivery of your drugs. If you live in a rural area or small town with few pharmacy choices, mail service can provide an attractive option.

If you have insurance or a discount card, be sure to include their mail service pharmacy on your list.

With some pharmacies, especially the larger chains (e.g., Walgreens.com, RiteAid.com, SamsClub.com), you can get the best of both worlds by shopping and ordering online and then picking up your drugs at the local store. Other chains operate Web pharmacies that are separate from their retail units, but they price similarly between the two, like Costco.com. At this writing, Wal-Mart does not reveal its drug prices on its website. If you live in one of the states listed in the following table, you can compare prices among competing pharmacies in your area. The prices tend to be out of date and the data sampling is irregular, but they can give you a good idea of which pharmacies in your area tend to offer the best deals.

Comparison shopping is worthwhile even if you have drug insurance or a drug discount card. You can

State Drug Price Comparison Websites

State	Website
Connecticut	http://www.cslib.org/attygenl/mainlinks/ tabindex20.htm
Florida	myfloridarx.com
Maine	http://www.maine.gov/dhhs/beas/drug_html/ drug_survey.htm
Maryland	http://www.oag.state.md.us/
Michigan	www.michigan.gov/mdch
Minnesota*	www.minnesotarxconnect.com
New Hamp.	http://www.egov.nh.gov/medicine-cabinet/
N. Mexico	http://www.ago.state.nm.us/know/know.htm
New York	http://www.nyagrx.org/
N. Dakota*	www.governor.state.nd.us/prescription-drug.html
Ohio	www.agrx.ag.state.oh.us
Vermont	http://www.atg.state.vt.us/display.php?smod=185
Washington	http://wa-bcm.com/drugprices/
W. Virginia	http://www.wvagrx.com/search.aspx
Wisconsin*	http://www.drugsavings.wi.gov/

*Canadian pharmacies only

often find retail pharmacy prices that are actually less than your insurance copayments or discount card prices. This is especially true for generic drugs. Some insurance plans require members to pay a $10 copayment for any generic drug prescription, even though the full retail price of such drugs is often much less than that. In those cases, you're better off not using your insurance or discount card, but always ask the price under both scenarios. For example, if you find that the retail price of your generic drug at one pharmacy is $6, but your drug insurance card requires a copayment of $10, don't use your card. But you have to ask the cash price before you'll know to do this.

Once you've assembled your pharmacy list, call each of the local ones and ask for their cash prices on each of your drugs in the quantities you want to buy, and enter them in the spreadsheet. Likewise, go to each of the Internet sites and do the same thing.

As discussed above, if you have a drug discount card, you will need to call the card issuer for the price. (Most pharmacies will not give you the discounted price over the phone.) Just call the telephone number on the back of your card and don't forget to ask about any quantity limitations.

STEP 4: EVALUATE AND DECIDE

Once you've surveyed the prices, total them up for each pharmacy and look at the results. If one of the pharmacies has the lowest prices for all of your drugs, then your decision is easy. Often, though, you'll find that the lowest total cost comes from a combination of two or more pharmacies. However, it's usually a good idea to obtain all your medications from the same pharmacy. That way, the pharmacist can easily run computerized drug interaction evaluations to make sure that none of your meds will combine in unintended ways to hurt you.

If one pharmacy has the lowest prices for all but one or two of your meds, call them back and ask if they will match the lowest price you found at another drugstore. Be sure to tell them if there are multiple prescriptions to be filled, and that you'd like to take all your business to them. This technique is most effective when the pharmacy has a policy of matching competitive prices. It can also help if the pharmacy is locally owned and you are a regular customer.

But if the price difference is still sufficient to make two or more pharmacies attractive, make sure that one of them has all of your drug information so that interactions can be checked. There are also online services that allow you to check for interactions yourself, but it's good to have a professional pharmacist do it, as she can then explain any risks that show up. This is no minor matter, as tens of thousands of people die or are injured each year because of unintended drug interactions.

STEP 5: MOVING PRESCRIPTIONS TO A NEW PHARMACY

There are two ways to move your current prescriptions to a new pharmacy. You can call your doctor's nurse to request the transfer, or you can ask your new pharmacy to do it for you. The latter is the easier course of action. Most retail and mail service pharmacies will be glad to take this task off your hands. After all, they do want your business.

All you have to do is provide your new pharmacy with the information off your current pill bottle (listed below), and they'll take care of it. Be sure to ask the pharmacy to request a higher quantity than the current prescription, if appropriate.

- Pharmacy name
- Pharmacy phone number
- Drug name/strength
- Prescription number (if you have it)
- Quantity (current and requested)
- Doctor's name
- Doctor's phone number

If you would rather call your doctor yourself for the prescription changes, go ahead. Again, don't forget to ask for the larger quantities. You will most likely speak to your doctor's nurse when you call, and she'll check with the doctor. The fastest way to get your new drugs is to ask that the new prescriptions be phoned in to your selected local pharmacies—after you've done your comparison shopping.

If you're going with an Internet or mail service pharmacy, ask your doctor for paper prescriptions, unless the pharmacy is specifically expecting it to be called in. Otherwise, there's a risk that the prescription might not get properly matched up with your ordering and shipping information. The pharmacy will tell you how to handle it. If you go with a paper script, most mail service pharmacies will require that you mail them the original. Faxes usually won't do, although some Canadian pharmacies may accept them (more on Canadian drugs in the next chapter).

STEP 6: GET NEW PRESCRIPTIONS IN WRITING

When a doctor prescribes a new drug for you or a family member, you usually have the option of getting it on paper or having his nurse phone it in to your pharmacy. Get the paper prescription. You can decide later where to purchase the drugs after you have had a chance to do your comparison shopping. If you ask for the prescription to be phoned in, you'll be passing up the opportunity to find the lowest cost pharmacy. When you get a paper prescription, make sure you understand what it says. Miserable doctor handwriting is cliché because it is so common. Make sure you can read it back to the doctor. Don't be embarrassed to ask him to explain the dosing instructions, which he will have written in a shorthand understood only by pharmacists. Besides facilitating comparison shopping, a clearly written prescription has the added benefit of reducing the risk that a pharmacist will accidentally give you the wrong drug and kill you—which happens at least 7,000 times a year in the U.S.[8]

If a prescription is for a maintenance medication to treat a long-term condition, like high blood pressure or cholesterol, you will want to buy the largest quantity you can afford (see above), but only after you know that you can tolerate the new drug and that it is effective. Many, many people have medicine cabinets full of obsolete drugs that they paid for but can't use. Avoid that particular waste of money.

If the prescribed med is a brand name drug, ask the doctor for enough samples to get you started; and ask for a written prescription for the larger quantities to buy after you know the drug works. Your doctor will usually write refillable prescriptions good for up to a year of continual treatment. Remember, your doctor will most likely not have samples for any generic drug you are taking, so if the new prescription is for a generic or for a brand name drug for which the doctor doesn't have samples, ask for two prescriptions: one for a short-term supply (15–30 days) to buy locally, and immediately, and the other for the larger supply after you do your comparison shopping.

If the new prescription is for an immediately needed drug, such as an antibiotic, pain medication, or antihistamine, you will be necessarily limited to buying it locally, at least initially. You want to begin taking it as soon as possible; so waiting for mail service delivery is not an option. That's another reason I keep a list of several local pharmacy phone numbers in my PDA. I then call each of them from my cell phone so I'll know where to buy it, even before I leave the doctor's parking lot. It still amazes me how much difference in prices I find when I make these calls.

STEP 7: REPEAT

When it comes time to refill an existing prescription, resist the temptation to simply call your current pharmacy to mail you a new batch. Drug prices change often, usually upward, and some pharmacies are slower than others at raising their prices. Also, drug wholesalers sometimes find themselves with excess inventories because they were able to get a particularly good deal from a drug manufacturer. Pharmacies will often take advantage of this to stock up at lower than normal prices, and then pass the savings on to their cash customers. Thus, you can often find unexpected bargains at one store but not another. Shop around.

Someday, we will be able to go online to virtually any pharmacy—retail or mail—and easily obtain complete, up-to-date pricing information. Until then, comparison shopping for drugs will require determination, personal ingenuity, and some inconvenience. After you've tried it, though, I predict you will be forever converted to the cause of price-savvy prescription drug buying. Happy hunting.

A SPECIAL NOTE ON INTERNET PHARMACIES

Let me put this to you gently. If you've been waiting to find a good reason to start using the Internet, finding lower cost prescription drugs is that reason. While this book will give you many useful ways to save money on your drugs without ever going online, nothing beats the Internet for access to quick, cheap (like free), important, up-to-date, money-saving information. It also makes ordering drugs from home delivery pharmacies much easier and much faster. If you don't have a computer, they are increasingly cheap and easy to use. If you don't want one or can't afford one, try your public library. Virtually every public library in the United States now offers free Internet access, as do many senior centers, relatives, or close friends.[9]

If you have never touched a computer, don't

worry. You won't need to know anything about how computers work. You'll just need someone to show you how to use the mouse and keyboard (trust me, it's easy), pull up the browser software (such as Microsoft Internet Explorer or Mozilla Firefox) and search engine (e.g., www.teoma.com, www.google.com, or www.yahoo.com), enter your search terms or destination website address, and off you go. You'll quickly pick up the rest and wonder why it took you so long to get around to it, and how quickly you picked it up when you did.

You'll need to exercise care in disclosing personal information on the Web. Many websites aren't covered by the federal HIPAA privacy statutes, and you don't want knowledge of your medical conditions to get around. When in doubt, read the website's online privacy policies; and if still in doubt, don't disclose private information.

Make sure you have top-rated virus and spyware protection on your computer, with regular online updates. Even then, you may find yourself researching a drug at several sites, only to receive unwanted spam e-mail within the hour trying to sell you the same drug.

Just because a pharmacy is on the Internet doesn't mean it is legitimate. Be careful. When it comes to pharmacies on the Web, you really need to separate the wheat from the chaff. Absolutely ignore unwanted spam e-mail messages pushing online pharmacies with unbelievable prices, and never order from any online pharmacy that doesn't require a doctor's prescription, especially those offering potent drugs promising to fix whatever needs fixing, reduce whatever needs reducing, or enlarge whatever needs enlarging. *DO NOT* switch or start any prescription medication without your doctor's agreement, despite the presence of online pharmacies offering prescription drugs without a prescription. When it comes to prescription drugs, *do not* self-diagnose, and *do not* self-prescribe. Personally, I never respond to spam come-ons. I figure the only thing I'll end up enlarging is my in-box of spam. Phony and un-regulated Internet pharmacies are also a major conduit of counterfeit drugs.

When buying online, purchase only government-approved drugs and only from properly licensed and regulated pharmacies. Make sure your preferred online pharmacies display their license information, and if in doubt, contact the relevant licensing authority to confirm.

Online pharmacies can save you money and, if that makes your drugs affordable, maybe even save your life. Just make sure you're dealing with reputable operations.

CHAPTER 12

Oh, Canada!

The importation of drugs from Canada and Europe has become a big issue in the United States in recent years. Many uninsured Americans have discovered they can buy most of their brand name drugs from Canadian pharmacies for about half the U.S. prices. As drug companies and the governments of the United States and Canada have erected barriers against this practice, consumers have begun to focus similar attention on other countries in Europe and elsewhere.[1,2,3] Regardless of the source, these people are engaging in a practice the Wall Street crowd calls arbitrage: buying something cheaper in one market, and then selling or consuming it in a higher priced market.

Canadian branded drugs have been cheaper than the same drugs in the U.S. for a long time, but remained largely unnoticed by anyone outside our northern tier states until two phenomena emerged: (1) painfully high U.S drug prices, and (2) the Internet. Nature abhors not only a vacuum, but huge price differentials for identical products, and the Internet made it easy for American consumers to take advantage of the differential instead of suffering from it. Arbitrage works.

In this chapter, I will address the following issues:

Why the Price Difference?

How Much Cheaper?

If It's Illegal, How Are So Many People Getting Away with It?

Is It Safe?

How Do I Buy Canadian Drugs?

Will They Accept My Doctor's Prescription?

How Long Will Delivery Take?

If you're not particularly interested in the economics, politics, law, and safety of importing Canadian drugs into the United States, you can skip down to "How Do I Buy Canadian Drugs?" and the subsequent related topics.

WHY THE PRICE DIFFERENCE?

Drugs in the U.S. are more expensive than in virtually every other country in the world—not just Canada. The U.S. is almost alone among industrialized countries in maintaining free-market economic policies for the pricing of healthcare products and services. The rest have imposed various versions of a single-payer, government-controlled system that regulates drug prices and fixes them at arbitrary levels. Without a free market in these countries, drug companies are faced with either selling their drugs for a much lower, government-imposed price, or not selling them at all. Even worse is the threat that any company not playing along will find its patents summarily revoked in those countries, thus allowing generic production by other companies. However, before you go writing to your congressperson to demand similar price controls, you should realize that it is the existence of the U.S. market that has allowed drug companies to invest many billions of dollars to create the vast array of life-enhancing, life-extending, and life-saving drugs that we so hate to pay for. I know we hear this argument a lot from the drug companies, but that doesn't make it wrong.

The problem for us is that the free-market policies on drug pricing in this country are up against even more powerful government policies that have entirely distorted the economics of health care into the increasingly unaffordable mess we have now (see Chapter 2). Our irrational system allows most consumers to remain both ignorant and indifferent about how much their drugs actually cost. This leaves the drug-sellers free to charge artificially high prices that insurance companies have little choice but to pay. If more Americans had to fork over all or a significant percentage of actual drug prices, we would all end up paying much lower prices than we do now. The power of motivated, savvy, price-conscious consumers could overnight force the brand name drug manufacturers to compete on the one factor they have thus far avoided: the price to the consumer. While Americans are increasingly concerned about U.S. drug prices, we are not yet at the tipping point where that concern is translated into drug company pricing strategies that look at the end-consumer as the price-sensitive customer making the key purchasing decision.

The drug manufacturers may complain about having to sell their drugs for less in other countries, but they cooperate in maintaining the system. They have long viewed the United States as their primary market. They have always known that they could safely invest hundreds of millions of dollars to develop a new drug, because the United States market would allow them to charge the insurance companies virtually anything they wanted in order to yield huge returns on that investment. The average insured consumer doesn't really care about individual drug prices, because he can still get any drug he needs by paying a copayment that has little or no direct relationship to that drug's price.

Foreign countries such as Canada have always been secondary markets for the drugmakers. They think of sales to these countries as the gravy on top of the United States' chicken-fried steak. Who cares if the Canadian, British, French, Italian, Chinese, Brazilian, and South African governments demand 50% or greater discounts from U.S. prices? The drugmakers are making a mint in the land of the expensive. And lest you think they are losing money in all those foreign countries, you should know they do very well selling their surplus production to these outlying, if somewhat annoying, markets. Once a drug is approved for sale and the factories are built, the actual cost of making additional pills is miniscule. Therefore, any price they can get in other countries that exceeds these low production costs goes directly to the bottom line. The high-priced American market ends up covering the drugmakers' development and marketing expenses. Thus, Americans, who make up only 5% of the world's population, pay 50% of the world's total drug bill.[4] We are heavily subsidizing the rest of the world's drug consumers.

The primary arguments by the drug companies in

support of the current system essentially boil down to these three: personal danger, economics, and insufficient capacity. All three of these arguments, in my opinion, are bogus.

The Danger Argument

This argument is that allowing consumers or pharmacies to import Canadian or European drugs would endanger us by exposing us to substandard, contaminated, non-approved, or counterfeit drugs. The FDA has repeatedly thrown up its hands and declared, "We cannot provide adequate assurance to the American public that the drug products delivered to consumers in the United States from foreign countries are the same products approved by the FDA."[5] This concern is a key reason often cited for the U.S. Congress's ban on drug imports by everyone *except* drug manufacturers. A more cynical explanation is suggested by the fact that more than $100 million is spent by drugmakers each year to influence senators and congresspeople with campaign contributions, lobbying, and issue advertising.[6]

I suggest that using the word "won't" instead of "cannot" in the above FDA statement would make it more truthful.

Implicit in the FDA statement is the notion that the FDA is unique among all the world's regulatory agencies in being able to protect its population from dangerous prescription drugs.

But if foreign drugs are so dangerous, why don't we see screaming headlines about tens of thousands of people dying daily in Canada, Europe, Asia, and Latin America from bad prescription drugs? The fact is that the other developed countries do a very good job of protecting their populations by regulating the safety and efficacy of their drugs. Canada's own regulatory agency, Health Canada, does a comparable job to the FDA's in that regard. Likewise, its provincial pharmacy regulatory agencies function similarly to our state boards of pharmacy to insure safe, professional pharmacy practices.[7] That's why Canadian and American consumers can be equally confident that their respective pharmacies will dispense safe, effective drugs.

The same goes for Europe. In fact, the fifteen original member countries of the European Union (EU) have allowed drug distributors to import lower cost drugs from other member countries for twenty-five years. Not only is this legal, but it is strongly encouraged as national policy in some EU countries. Some high-cost EU countries are estimated to import as much as 20% of their brand name drugs this way. A recent study of this system by AARP found no significant problems and *no* documented instances of counterfeiting arising from the practice. It seems that the European regulators have successfully and proactively been able to assure their citizens of the safety of imported drugs from approved sources, something the FDA says it "cannot" do.[8]

Some may point to a recent study of 1,009 online "Canadian" pharmacies as proof that Canadian pharmacies are dangerous. It reported that only 214 of this number were actually located in Canada, with the rest actually being in other countries. This, of course, says nothing about the quality of actual Canadian pharmacies, but conveys boatloads about the need for care in purchasing drugs through any Internet website claiming to be a pharmacy.

Many, including this author, believe that our government has failed American consumers who want to buy less expensive pharmaceuticals from other countries. It has refused to work with international drug regulators to develop common standards for the safety and effectiveness of drugs and dispensing, regardless of location of buyer and seller. If they did, drugs meeting those standards could flow across borders as easily as food and automobiles do now, and we could have a worldwide market of buyers and sellers enforcing rational, fair pricing.

The Economics Argument

Here's the economic argument as put forth by James K. Glassman and John R. Lott, Jr., in an op-ed piece in the Wall Street Journal: "If U.S. spending on drugs dropped sharply—as a result of re-importation—drug companies would simply stop making new drugs.[9] Re-importation, which, at first glance, seems like a decent idea, would be a disaster for all concerned." This is the sort of steady-state argument that reminds me of H. L. Mencken's aphorism, "For every human problem, there is a neat, simple solution; and it is always wrong."[10] In the case of the op-edsters, they assume that the drug companies would continue business as usual in the face of legal drug imports, except that they would "simply" stop inventing new drugs. I suggest that there are a few other things they would try first, such as streamlining their bloated, bureaucratic cost structures; rationalizing their cost accounting and pricing models; lobbying the government to help them enforce their patents internationally; and engaging in tougher negotiations with foreign governments that insist on a free ride. Cutting off research and development, their life's blood, would be one of the *last* things they would do.

In my opinion, you don't need to pay any more attention to this argument than you would if the General Motors Corporation demanded that you should be willing to pay more for a Chevrolet than an equivalent Toyota just because GM's workers have higher healthcare and retirement costs. The essence of consumerism is that you should be able to decide for yourself whether you're willing to pay more or whether you just want the best car for the lowest price. Same for your drugs.

The Insufficient Capacity Argument

The idea here is that, if 300 million Americans could legally import drugs from Canada, then that small country would be overwhelmed by our demand, especially if the drug companies intensified their current practices of limiting drug exports to Canada to choke off the return trade. The poor Canadians themselves could suffer crippling drug shortages. In fact, some Canadian officials are beginning to buy this argument themselves, and are proposing to eliminate the export of drugs to U.S. consumers.

This is another steady-state argument that assumes there won't be pharmacies in yet other well-regulated countries that will happily step in to satisfy U.S. demand. In fact this is already happening, with Web-based pharmacies cropping up in the U.K., Ireland, and other countries. The drug companies may be able to choke off supply to one small country, but not to the entire world. The argument also assumes that the drug companies would willingly continue to sell to foreign countries at significantly lower prices than the U.S. In the face of substantial re-importation, they might instead decide to adopt worldwide pricing structures. Finally, it assumes that the drug companies would stick to their current U.S. pricing model that provides big rebates and discounts to drug distributors, but none to the ultimate consumer—especially the uninsured consumer. Perhaps the drug companies might instead find it advantageous to adopt a free-market, consumer-driven business model (just like virtually every other industry in the United States) that focuses on providing their customers with the best drugs at the lowest prices. They might have to work harder for their profits, but they *would* work harder for their profits, and consumers would finally get their doctors to work with them to make their purchasing decisions on the basis of quality *and* price.

HOW MUCH CHEAPER?

Canadian brand name drugs are usually 40–60% cheaper than the same or equivalent drugs sold in the United States. However, many of the low-income Americans who are buying Canadian drugs are probably unaware that they can qualify for one or more patient assistance programs in the United States that can deliver the same drugs for free (see Chapter 10: "Free and Discounted Drug Programs"). The Canadian pharmacies cannot beat free. In addition, the new 2006 Medicare drug benefit provides U.S. drugs to our senior and disabled citizens at essentially Canadian prices.

Finally, savvy consumers buying in the United States can often find drug prices that are comparable to Canada's. One example is the antidepressant drug Zoloft, which is available in tablet form in the U.S., but only as capsules in Canada. You can split Zoloft tablets, but you can't split capsules. So if you are taking 50 mg of Zoloft once a day, you can buy 100 mg tablets and split them in the U.S., but you can only buy 50 mg capsules from Canada—at about the same price as the tablet-split doses here. Thus, there is no savings from Canada, and you don't have to worry about border customs delays for the American drugs.

Generic drugs in the United States are usually less expensive than the same generics in Canada, especially if you use the savvy shopping techniques in Chapter 11.[11] For generic drugs, there's not much reason to think about Canada.

However, there are some generic drugs available in Canada that are not yet allowed in the United States. For example, generic versions of Zoloft (for depression) and Pravachol (for cholesterol) are available in Canada but not the U.S. For these drugs, buying from Canada can provide a double dose of savings.

So genuine Canadian drugs may in fact save you a lot of money, but only if:

1. You are uninsured.
2. You need brand name drugs.
3. You don't qualify for an American patient assistance program.

IF IT'S ILLEGAL, HOW ARE SO MANY PEOPLE GETTING AWAY WITH IT?

According to the FDA, virtually all drugs imported from Canada violate federal law, because they are unapproved, incorrectly labeled, or dispensed without a valid prescription.[12] Despite this, the FDA pretty much turns a blind eye to people who import for their own use. There have been some border seizures of consumer-bound meds, but only in token amounts. The FDA explains their policy as follows: "[U]nder FDA's Personal Importation policy, as a matter of enforcement discretion in certain defined circumstances, FDA allows consumers to import otherwise illegal drugs. However, this policy is non intended [sic] to allow importation of foreign versions of drugs of which there is a FDA-approved version. Moreover, the policy simply describes the agency's enforcement priorities. It does not change the law, and it does not give a license to persons to import or export illegal drugs into the United States."[13]

In other words, the FDA confirms that importation is illegal; that they don't approve of it; that they aren't enforcing the law; and that they can change their minds at any time. My guess is that they will not change their minds; at least not until the new Medicare drug benefit takes full effect in 2006. It also depends on whether the AARP loses interest in the issue. Since there is no AAUP (American Association of Uninsured Persons) to take up the lobbying slack, things could change.

The enforcement issue is a different story if you're an American trying to make a buck from Canadian drug imports. The FDA has warned that anyone who helps others to obtain imported drugs could "be found civilly and criminally liable," and it has gone after commercial operations in the United States that were attempting to do just that.[14,15]

As long as you import limited quantities for your own use, you probably will not be hassled by the FDA, but there are no guarantees. They could change their "enforcement discretion" at any time. Just realize that you will be breaking the law. But so do all those people who pass me on the interstate after I've set my cruise control on the speed limit.

IS IT SAFE?

The FDA's stated position on safety is clear: "FDA is very concerned about the safety risks associated with the importation of prescription drugs from foreign countries. In our experience, many drugs obtained from foreign sources that purport and appear to be the same as U.S.-approved prescription drugs have been of unknown quality. We cannot provide adequate assurance to the American public that the drug products delivered to consumers in the United States from foreign countries are the same products approved by FDA."[16] Since the FDA's position is essentially that all foreign drugs are per se not approvable, this last statement is like saying, "We won't permit anything brown to be imported, because brown things aren't allowed [by us]."

They cite instances of non-approved, suspect, understrength, overstrength, contaminated, or outright counterfeit drugs from bogus pharmacies. Unfortunately, the FDA has not broken out statistics between the merely non-approved drugs (technically all Canadian drugs) and the truly bad ones. One gets the impression that the FDA is not going to say anything balanced, much less positive about the subject. Period. They are providing no consumer guidance at all, other than recommending that consumers not import drugs.

As discussed above, Canada's and Europe's regulation of drug safety, effectiveness, and dispensing is on a par with the United States'. If you walk into a

Canadian or European retail pharmacy, you can have a high degree of confidence that the drugs you receive there are as safe and effective as the drugs you can buy at an American pharmacy.

The problem, as I mentioned earlier, is that a large majority of "Canadian" Internet pharmacies aren't actually located in Canada. A recent investigation of 1,009 online "Canadian" pharmacies found that only 214 of them were located in Canada.[17] Evidence indicated that 85% of the rest are in the United States, and the remainder in other countries, including Vietnam and the Czech Republic. Since it is extremely unlikely that the U.S. pharmacies are able to offer legitimate drugs at Canadian prices, there is a strong suspicion that they are selling stolen or counterfeit medications; and that they aren't really pharmacies at all. This is serious stuff and strongly supports the notion that you must know your supplier before buying anything from them.

In the wake of FDA's unhelpfulness, several states have become proactive in recognizing the reality of drug importation, and in providing consumer information and guidance to help minimize risks and lower costs. Some are actively aiding and abetting the purchase of Canadian and English drugs by their employees and citizens. According to Illinois Governor Rod Blagojevich, "The federal government has failed to act. So it's time that we do."[18]

In 2004, Minnesota became the first state to provide financial incentives for state employees to purchase their prescription drugs from Canadian pharmacies.[19] They have a website to route Minnesota residents (or anyone else) to pre-screened Canadian and U.K. pharmacies. They sent pharmacy investigators to visit eight

Canadian candidate pharmacies for possible inclusion in the program, of which only two passed their scrutiny.[20] Since then, the states of Illinois, Kansas, Missouri, North Dakota, Rhode Island, Vermont, Wisconsin, and Nevada have added similar sites or plan to.[21] Given the FDA's abdication of any active quality-assurance role, these state efforts comprise the nearest thing to a Good Housekeeping seal of approval to be found for Canadian and U.K. Internet pharmacies. The states' websites are listed later in this chapter. Note: the FDA has limited its role to sending warnings to the offending states, and has not yet moved to shut down any of them.[22]

Highlighting the need for consumers to exercise great care in picking a Canadian pharmacy, Minnesota's investigators found numerous flaws in the six Internet pharmacies that failed to pass muster.[23] These included understaffing of professional pharmacists, inadequate supervision of production technicians, and substandard storage of temperature-sensitive drug inventory. All can significantly raise the risk of your receiving incorrect or otherwise harmful medications.

So what should you do? I'm not completely comfortable telling you to break the law and buy Canadian drugs—although I must admit I've done it myself. The upshot is this: if you buy from a legitimate, physical, licensed pharmacy that is actually in Canada, then Canada's regulatory oversight process provides assurance that the pharmacy will sell you safe and effective drugs. However, you will be in legal limbo, with neither Health Canada nor the FDA accepting any responsibility if something goes wrong.

HOW DO I BUY CANADIAN DRUGS?

There are two ways to get cheap Canadian drugs. One is to travel to Canada and have your prescription filled at a Canadian retail pharmacy, after getting a Canadian doctor to endorse your U.S. prescription. As I said above, this is the safest way to obtain Canadian drugs. While hardly practical for most of us, many Americans do just that—especially those living in the Northern states. Organized bus tours have disgorged them by the thousands into the arms of welcoming, legitimate pharmacies.

The second way is to order from an Internet-based mail service pharmacy. I've already pointed out how risky this is if you're not dealing with a legitimate, licensed, regulated, law-abiding, truly Canadian-based pharmacy.

For starters, absolutely ignore and delete any unsolicited spam e-mails advertising "Canadian" pharmacies. Otherwise, you may find your "drugs" arriving from India, Thailand, or Vietnam. A maple leaf logo and low prices do not a Canadian pharmacy make.

For several years, I purchased prescription medications for my family and myself from Hillhurst Clinical Pharmacy (formerly Grace Clinical Pharmacy) in Calgary, Alberta (www.gracemeds.com; telephone 1-866-301-3784; fax 1-866-601-3784). I have met in the U.S. with one of the principals of the company and have spoken by telephone on several occasions with another. I have found them to be a reliable, trustworthy operation. An American doctor friend of mine visited them a few years ago, and returned praising it as one of the best run, most professional pharmacies she had ever seen. Because of my personal experience with them and my friend's (informal, but informed) recommendation, Hillhurst is the only Canadian website with a linkage at www.HydeRx.com. I have no financial or other beneficial dealings with them other than my occasional personal purchase of their low cost medications. Nonetheless, I do not have sufficient professional knowledge to recommend them outright. I'm just telling you about my own experience.

I mentioned above that Minnesota had sent investigators to evaluate pharmacies for inclusion in that state's referral website. Of these, only one, Total Care Pharmacy in Calgary, Alberta, "far surpassed the other seven in many aspects of overall pharmacy practice."[24] In the end, Minnesota decided to list two of the pharmacies on its website, Total Care and Granville Pharmacy in Vancouver, B.C. Since then, they have added the option of ordering United Kingdom–sourced drugs, as well. Some brand name drugs have become scarce at Canadian Web pharmacies because of restricted shipments by U.S. drug companies in an attempt to cut off the cross-border trade. I personally cannot vouch for any of these international pharmacies, although I did use Total Care a few years ago, and found their service to be satisfactory.

If you decide to purchase Canadian drugs, here are the state-sponsored websites I mentioned above. Of these, Minnesota's appears to be the most sophisticated, although these things tend to change quickly on the Internet. These state sites are probably the closest thing you'll find in this country to official government approval of Canadian drug importing.

State	Website
Illinois	http://www.i-saverx.net/
Kansas	http://www.accesskansas.org/healthykansasrx/isaverx.shtml
Minnesota	http://www.minnesotarxconnect.com/
Missouri	http://www.i-saverx.net/about.htm
N. Dakota	http://governor.state.nd.us/prescription-drug.html
Vermont	http://www.ahs.state.vt.us/ISaveRXVT.cfm
Wisconsin	http://drugsavings.wi.gov/news_detail.asp?onid=42&locid=2

WILL THEY ACCEPT MY DOCTOR'S PRESCRIPTION?

Any legitimate Canadian pharmacy will not directly honor a prescription from any doctor who is not licensed in Canada. Instead, the pharmacy will arrange for a Canadian-licensed physician to review your doctor's prescription and the health information you enter on the pharmacy's website, and then endorse it if she finds it to be appropriate. When I went through this initial process with Hillhurst, they referred my prescription to a dual-licensed physician practicing in the United States. I received a telephone call from someone in his office to clarify and confirm my medical history and drug allergies before issuance of a Canada-legal script. The process was professional, thorough, and easy.

The Canadian government itself has threatened to interrupt cross-border drug sales by making it illegal for Canadian doctors to cosign any prescription without first having examined the patient, presumably physically.[25] Such a move could effectively shut down the entire consumer retail drug export industry in Canada, although there appears to be no shortage of other countries' pharmacies ready to rush in and fill the gap.

HOW LONG WILL DELIVERY TAKE?

Once the pharmacy has a Canada-legal prescription, they should be able to ship your drugs within a day or two, assuming they have it in inventory. Some drugs have become scarce, as some U.S.-based drug companies forbid distribution of their products through any pharmacy that exports to the U.S., so it could take longer.

Once shipped, your drugs will have to clear U.S. Customs at the border. This can sometimes add several days to your shipment. Make sure you order refills in plenty of time to avoid running out. It is unlikely that your drugs will be seized by border inspectors, but it has happened on rare occasions. If it happens to you, you will have no recourse to anyone for your loss.

Brand name drugs from Canada can be a real bargain, but only if you do your homework, find the right pharmacy, and don't mind breaking this particular law. Good hunting and good luck.

CHAPTER 13

SPECIAL SENIOR REPORT:
Medicare Part D
Prescription Drug Coverage

THE MEDICARE MODERNIZATION
ACT OF 2003

When Medicare was created in 1965 to provide health benefits for disabled and elderly Americans, it had no prescription drug benefit. This wasn't a big deal at the time, since prescription drugs did not have the widespread role they have now in treating and preventing disease—particularly chronic disease. They also weren't very expensive. Since then, the lack of a Medicare drug benefit has become a costly burden to millions of people who have been completely at the mercy of extremely high and continually rising drug costs. At least 10 million Medicare beneficiaries had no drug coverage in 2005. Many of the additional millions were fortunate enough to have supplemental Medigap or Medicare Advantage (formerly Medicare + Choice) drug coverage, but they have experienced rising costs and increasing limits on coverage. Even the millions more with private retirement coverage from their former employers have seen their benefits dramatically eroded to the point where they worry about whether they will ultimately have any benefits at all.

This picture changed dramatically beginning in 2003, when Congress passed the Medicare Prescription Drug Improvement and Modernization Act of 2003. Usually referred to as the Medicare Modernization Act, or simply MMA, it, for the first time, created an insurance-style Medicare prescription drug benefit to be offered to all 42 million Medicare beneficiaries.

If you are, or soon will be, eligible for Medicare, you need to know about this coverage, and particularly about the choices you will be required to make. While it is a completely voluntary program, it is critically important that you make the effort to learn your options. The cost of doing nothing at the right time could be financially disastrous to you when the wrong time rolls around.

The MMA also provided for two interim programs, a Medicare-approved drug discount card program and the Medicare Replacement Drug Demonstration program, both of which end in late 2005 or in early 2006, so I will not cover these, other than to briefly summarize later.

Below, I will first give you a primer on the new Medicare program itself, followed by specific recommendations to make sure you make the right decisions to maximize your benefit. If you elect to participate in this drug benefit, you will find that most of the techniques I have discussed for saving money elsewhere in this book will be just as applicable for you as they were before this new coverage became available.

Medicare Prescription Drug Plans

Since November 15, 2005, all of Medicare's 42 million beneficiaries have been able to sign up for Medicare Part D prescription drug coverage that works like regular commercial drug insurance. Key features of this program are as follows.

Government Regulated

The federal government's Centers for Medicare & Medicaid Services (CMS) is charged with regulating MMA, and has issued approximately 2000 pages of regulations to specify how MMA will be implemented and operated.

Privately Administered

The MMA requires that it consist almost exclusively of competing private plans, rather than a single government plan where bureaucrats manage drug benefits, set prices, or decide which drugs would be covered. To date, many private insurers and pharmacy-benefit companies have responded with offerings, and every eligible American will have a choice of at least eleven competing plans, with some having as many as twenty-three plans to choose from.

Replaces Interim Drug Discount Card Program

MMA provided for an interim drug discount card program that was to be a temporary stopgap to assist Medicare beneficiaries with their drug costs before the Medicare drug benefit began on January 1, 2006. This program allowed private organizations to sponsor drug discount cards that met certain Medicare requirements. These cards, which cost no more than $30 per year, were available from May 2004 until December 31, 2005. If you currently hold such a card, you can use it until May 15, 2006, or until you join a Medicare prescription drug plan, whichever occurs first. After that, you will not be able to use or renew your discount card.

Replaces Temporary Medicare Replacement Drug Demonstration

This program ran from September 2004 through December 31, 2005. It allowed up to 50,000 Medicare beneficiaries with life-threatening diseases to obtain coverage for certain expensive home-administered drugs instead of having to have comparable treatments only in doctors' offices.

Average Savings About 50%

The Congressional Budget Office has estimated that the average beneficiary will save $465 on his drug costs during the first year, including all premiums, deductibles, copayments, and coverage gaps. This amount is estimated to represent a savings of about 50% on average—somewhat less than the amount I expect most people to be able to save with this book. If, by using the principles in this book, you can cut your drug costs in half, then Medicare may be able to let you cut them by *another* 50%. That would be a terrific one-two punch for your drug budget.

MAJOR COST AND COVERAGE PROVISIONS

The Medicare Part D drug benefit can be a mystifying program, subject to interminable regulations, opaque definitions, confusing benefits, seemingly infinite choices, and befuddling exceptions; all engendering uncertainty about what you should do. I'll try to guide you through some of the shoals, and please bear in mind that *this is important!* Please don't ignore this opportunity; it could cost you dearly in the future.

Let's start with a summary overview of MMA's salient features.

Information to Support Your Decisions

The government announced in early 2005 that it would spend $300 million during that year to try to educate the 42 million Medicare beneficiaries who are eligible for the benefit.

If you receive printed information from the government on this program, take the time to read it. You can call their toll-free hotline (1-800-MEDICARE) with questions about what you've read, heard, feared, or suspected. I don't know how reliable this telephone advice will be, but if it's anything like the IRS, make sure that you verify anything you hear that's important.

If you utilize the Internet, go to www.medicare.gov and www.cms.hhs.gov/map/map.asp for extensive information on the program. If you're not on the Internet, I strongly recommend that you find someone to help you get on it, as this website can help you narrow your decision choices based on your own prescription drug history. In addition to fact sheets and more detailed publications, you will be able to complete your own specific customized worksheets on premiums, covered drugs, your current drug costs, pharmacies, pharmacy services, and other important features of your drug plan choices. It may not always be the easiest site to navigate, but it is better than most and very much worth the effort. Just be patient, and you'll get the hang of it.

If you would like individualized assistance, you can contact your local State Health Insurance Assistance Program (SHIP). This program has counselors in every state and several U.S. territories that are available to provide free one-on-one help with your Medicare questions or problems. You can locate contact information for your local SHIP offices at http://www.medicare.gov/contacts/static/allStateContacts.asp or by calling 1-800-MEDICARE.

You can also get one-on-one help from the Access to Benefits Coalition, which has a partnership arrangement with CMS (the Medicare administrative agency). Contact them for information on a local agency that can help you:

The Access to Benefits Coalition
300 D Street SW, Suite 801
Washington, DC 20024
Phone: 202-479-6670
Fax: 202-479-0735
info@accesstobenefits.org

Eligibility

If you are eligible for Medicare, then you are eligible for Medicare Part D (D for drug) benefit. I emphasize *eligible*, because you will not be automatically enrolled, *unless* you are one of about 6 million

Medicare beneficiaries with very low income or are in a nursing home. If you do not fall into these categories, you will have to decide if you want to participate in Medicare Part D. And if you do, which of the myriad, differing, confusing, competing private plans offering a variety of qualifying Rx benefits in your area will you join and pay for?

Later, I'll provide more guidance on how to more easily navigate this decision process.

Medigap Policies

After January 1, 2006, there is no reason for you to continue with any Medigap drug policy that you may currently have, although you may do so. If you do decide to continue with Medigap, you will have to pay the full premium cost, which is usually more than $120 per month. If, instead, you drop the Medigap policy and buy Part D coverage, your premium will cost you, on average, only about $32.20 a month and, in many cases, much less. Also, the Part D coverage will almost certainly have better catastrophic protection. If you don't have Medigap drug coverage now, you will no longer be able to purchase it. Insurers will be able to continue to issue Medigap policies without drug coverage to supplement Medicare Parts A and B hospital and outpatient coverage.

Again, the worst thing you can do is nothing. I apologize if I sound alarmist, but I want to emphasize the importance of this issue. Pay attention, use the tools available to you, and make an informed decision.

Enrollment

Enrollment for Part D began November 15, 2005, for current Medicare eligibles. The Part D reg-

ulations specify three different kinds of enrollment
periods

1. **The initial enrollment period.** If you are eligible
   for Part D as of November 15, 2005, you will
   have from then until May 15, 2006, to enroll in
   a Part D plan. If you become eligible later, then
   your initial enrollment period will be similar to
   the one established for Medicare Part B (i.e.,
   Medicare's optional medical insurance that covers doctors and hospital outpatient services).

2. **The annual coordinated election period.** This
   is the period once a year during which you can
   elect to change to another Part D plan. It will
   normally be from November 15 through December 31 each year; but the first one that began November 15, 2005, will be extended
   through May 15, 2006, in order to sign up as
   many people as possible.

3. **Special enrollment periods.** Essentially, CMS,
   the federal agency that administers Medicare,
   has left itself the flexibility to respond to special circumstances to offer additional enrollment periods, such as for changes in residence
   or other factors. I suggest that you don't count
   on this catchall to kick in if you don't get
   around to making the right decision for yourself during the normal enrollment periods.

Premiums

There will be a monthly premium for drug coverage. If you are a typical beneficiary, you will pay 25%

of the premium, and the government will pay the remaining 75%. An individual's share is estimated to average about $32.20 per month. However, this can vary by plan, with some costing $20 per month or less. If you are poor, you will not be required to pay this premium.

Penalty for Failure to Timely Enroll

Once you are eligible to enroll in Part D, I suggest that you don't delay your decision. If you fail to maintain what CMS calls creditable prescription drug coverage for a period of sixty-three days, then you will be subject to a late enrollment penalty in the form of higher premiums than you would otherwise have to pay. This could get expensive over time.

Examples of creditable coverage may include:[1]

- Coverage under a prescription drug plan or Medicare Advantage plan with prescription drug coverage
- Medicaid
- Group health plan
- State Pharmaceutical Assistance Program
- VA coverage
- Medigap with prescription drug coverage
- Military service-related coverage, including TRICARE

If you are eligible for Medicare, ask your employer or health plan if your current drug coverage meets the requirement for creditable coverage. If it does not, then you should consider dropping it and signing up for a Medicare Part D drug coverage plan now; if you do it later, you could have to pay a penalty.

How much is the penalty? It's hard to say at this point. The regulations call for it to be the *greater of* 1% of the *base beneficiary premium* for each uncovered month *or* "an amount that CMS determines is actuarially sound for each uncovered month . . ."[2] A "special rule" for 2006 and 2007 sets the penalty at 1% for each uncovered month unless the secretary specifies another amount. Your guess is as good as mine as to what the difference is between the normal rule and the special rule. They sound pretty much the same.

In any event, the definition of *base beneficiary premium* is very bureaucratic and murky. Until it is clarified, you should assume that the penalty will indeed be punitive. Their goal is to prevent healthy people from gaming the system and waiting until they need the coverage to sign up. If enough people actually do this, you can reasonably expect CMS to calculate the actual cost of such "adverse selection" and to establish an "actuarially sound" amount that is considerably more painful than the 1% per month rule.

If you're eligible for coverage now, don't count on still being able to get it later at a cost you can afford.

Subsidies

The Congressional Budget Office has estimated that about a third of all Medicare beneficiaries are eligible for low-income subsidies. These subsidies reduce or eliminate premiums, deductibles, copayments, and coverage gaps. Here's a breakdown of the eligibility groups for these additional subsidies.

DUAL MEDICARE/MEDICAID ELIGIBLES—FULL SUBSIDY

About 6 million individuals who are now covered by both Medicare and Medicaid are automatically enrolled in Part D and provided the full subsidy. There are another 1 million or so who are eligible, but who have not previously enrolled in Medicaid, and will need to do so to obtain the full subsidy. All of these Part D dual enrollees will pay no premium, have no deductible, and their copayments will be as little as $1 for generic drugs and $3 for brand drugs.

UNDER 135% OF POVERTY LINE

About 3 million Medicare beneficiaries are not eligible for Medicaid, but have limited assets and incomes that are less than 135% of the poverty level. If they can successfully navigate the seven-page (!) government application *and* sign up for Part D coverage, then Medicare will cover about 96% of their drug costs. If you know someone in this category, I suggest you go out of your way to tactfully help him or her get the necessary assistance to secure this coverage.

135–150% OF POVERTY LINE

About 1.6 million beneficiaries in this category (and with limited assets) will pay a sliding-scale premium and copayments of only 15% of their drug costs, but only if they, too, can wade through the seven-page application and also sign up for Part D coverage. They need your help, too, so please refer them to one of the agencies listed above.

"LIMITED ASSETS"

The asset test for the above subsidies will count only liquid assets and real estate holdings *other than* your home or farm (if you live on it). Nonliquid assets, such as "wedding rings, family heirlooms, and burial plots" will not be counted (http://www.cms. hhs.gov/medicarereform/pdbma/fs-pdbmafinalrules. pdf). However, if you are on Medicaid, be warned that your state can bill your estate after you die for the costs of your Medicaid-paid care.[3]

Benefits

Here is a summary of the basic benefits for the approximately two-thirds of the 42 million eligibles who do not receive subsidies and who pay their full 25% premium contribution.

ANNUAL DEDUCTIBLE

Enrollees will pay 100% of the first $250 of covered drug expenses during each year, although many plans have a zero deductible.

COINSURANCE AFTER THE DEDUCTIBLE

After the $250 annual deductible is met, the enrollee will pay 25% of the next $2,000 of allowable drug costs during the current benefit year (i.e., up to $2,250 in total costs). Many plans replace this requirement with fixed-dollar copayments.

THE DOUGHNUT HOLE

After an enrollee has incurred $2250 in total drug costs and thus paid $750 out of pocket during the current benefit year ($250 deductible plus the maximum coinsurance of $500), he will then have to pay 100% of the next $2,850, the so-called doughnut hole. This means that he is personally liable for a total of $3,600 out of the first $5,100 in total drug costs each year. These costs are in addition to the average monthly premium of approximately $32.20. Some plans offer additional coverage for the doughnut hole, with some covering generic drugs only.

COVERAGE AFTER THE DOUGHNUT HOLE

For any total drug costs in excess of $5,100, the enrollee will pay 5% and the government the remaining 95%. One of the benefits of Part D coverage is that there is no maximum amount on your coverage. Some private plans place maximum limits on how much of your drug costs they will cover on an annual and/or lifetime basis. Despite the doughnut hole, Part D offers a level of catastrophic coverage rarely, if ever, seen in the private insurance world. On the other hand, private insurance normally has much better non-catastrophic benefits and no Doughnut Hole.

TROOP SPENDING

The part that the beneficiary pays for deductibles, coinsurance, and doughnut holes is called out-of-pocket spending. The feds have invented an acronym called True Out-Of-Pocket (TROOP) spending. They have defined it in such a way that allows for a variety of third party payments to count as legitimate out-of-pocket spending on your behalf, as though you had spent it yourself. Thus a charitable organization might contribute to an enrollee's cost, as might the state or another individual. If a beneficiary has a health spending account, such as an HRA (Health Reimbursement Arrangement),

HSA (Health Savings Account), or FSA (Flexible Spending Account), then expenditures from these can also count as allowable TROOP spending.

SUPPLEMENTAL DRUG COVERAGE IN ADDITION TO BASIC PART D COVERAGE

Those who can sign up for a full-coverage Medicare Advantage plan (formerly called Medicare + Choice) from a managed care organization may be able to pay lower copayments than under standard Part D, avoid the deductible, and even avoid the Doughnut Hole. However, the premium will be higher and there may be more coverage restrictions for some drugs than for a basic Medicare drug plan. In order for a plan sponsor to provide a more expensive "higher option" drug coverage plan as part of a Medicare Advantage program, it must also offer *either* a basic Part D plan *or* a drug plan that includes supplemental coverage but costs no more than the basic Part D coverage. If you can afford supplemental coverage, it's worthwhile to analyze how much your known drug needs will cost you, including premiums.

COVERED DRUGS

Before signing up for a particular Part D plan, be sure to check that it will cover the drugs you are currently taking. It may not. Plans are allowed to adopt an allowable drug list, called a formulary, which can restrict an enrollee's access to certain drugs. If your drugs aren't on the formulary list, you could be required either to pay their entire cost or to have your doctor change your medications in order to receive coverage. While you can appeal such limitations on the basis of medical necessity, you will need a doctor's certification and be prepared to endure the plan's appeal procedures.

E-Prescribing

Participating drug plans will be required to support electronic prescribing by doctors, although this will be voluntary for physicians and pharmacies. To the extent that this encourages doctors to use electronic information systems to help you get the drugs you need at the lowest possible cost, it will be a good thing. So will any reduction in prescribing and dispensing mistakes from sloppy handwriting.

Grievances and Appeals Procedures

Plans are required to establish a process for hearing and resolving enrollees' grievances in a timely manner, and to maintain records on the number of grievances they process. In general, the procedures governing grievances, coverage determinations, redeterminations, reconsiderations, and appeals are the same as those that apply to the Medicare Advantage program. There are five levels of appeals procedures. Five!

One new feature of the appeals procedure is worth noting. For enrollees who exhaust the normal administrative appeal procedures with Medicare staff, there has long been a procedure where the enrollee can present her case before an impartial administrative law judge. There have been 283,000 such hearings and decisions during the past few years, with fully two-thirds of them resulting in decisions against the Medicare bureaucrats.[4] A recent change in the process, however, will pretty much do away with face-to-face hearings between judges and enrollees, and will replace them with video teleconference links. The intent is both to make the judges more productive and to allow the Medicare beneficiaries to have easier and more local access to video hearing facilities than previously available through fewer than three hearing locations per state. The secretary of the U.S. Department of Health and Human Services has promised "vastly more access points."[5] So far, this sounds pretty good, but it has been a controversial decision, with fears that Medicare officials will have an unfair advantage against beneficiaries who may be uncomfortable with the technology and unable to be properly seen and assessed by the judge. The rules are new, so it is too early to see how it really works out. My bet is that both sides have a point, and the process will have to be tweaked to get it right.

WHAT TO MAKE OF PART D?

If I may I editorialize for a moment on the new Medicare Part D program, I have to say that I like it. I think is was intelligently designed to provide much-needed financial relief for seniors and the disabled while providing strong incentives for enrollees to continue to be price savvy drug shoppers. Without such incentives that actually work, the program would run the substantial risk of pricing itself out of the market, as continued double-digit drug inflation doubles costs every five years. Thank goodness it does not mandate fixed dollar copayments (which you'll see anyway from many health plan Part D offerings) that could prove financially disastrous for the program. The various layers of deductibles and coinsurance assure that the basic benefit members will have strong incentives to minimize their drug costs while paying affordable premiums. Nice trick.

I also like the fact that the program has successfully encouraged so many private plans to compete for your business on the basis of strong benefits and low premiums. Just check out www.cms.hhs.gov/map/map.asp to find a convenient summary of all the plans being offered in your state. In many states, you can find basic benefit premiums for less than $10 per month. You can often find other plans that eliminate both the deductible and the doughnut hole for those willing to pay higher premiums.

HOW TO DECIDE

Buried in the Part D regulations and supporting documents is the statement, "CMS will establish a comprehensive set of activities to broadly disseminate information about Part D coverage to individuals who are eligible or prospectively eligible for Part D benefits. This will include developing a price comparison tool, similar to the price comparison tool currently available for Medicare-approved discount drug cards."[6]

Brace yourself. In the span of a single page, I'm about to say *two* nice things about Medicare Part D and CMS. The first was the above opinion about the benefit. The second is this: I really liked the custom price comparison tool on the Medicare website for the old discount drug card program. It provided a relatively easy way to sort through the scores of competing drug cards and find the one plan that could save the most money for each individual.

You could just type in the drugs you were taking and the amount you were paying and it would then list the discount cards available in your area by how much you could save on each. Very simple and very cool. If they succeed in porting this tool over to Part D coverage, finding the best plan for you will be greatly simplified.

Here's what I suggest you do.

1. **Take inventory.** Go to your medicine cabinet and take out all the medications you are currently taking.

2. **Research prices.** How much did you have to pay for these? If you don't have records, call the pharmacy that dispensed them and ask how much you'd have to pay now (i.e., before the Part D benefit).

3. **Go to www.medicare.gov.** Navigate your way to the Part D price comparison tool.

4. **Answer the questions.** You will need to provide some basic information, including your zip code and a promise that you won't sue anyone if the pricing information on the site turns out to be wrong.

5. **Enter your drugs.** Enter the data from steps 1 and 2, and click to proceed.

6. **View your plan options and decide.** Compare the results of your analysis to see which plan of-

fers you the best net benefits, after including any premiums, deductibles, coinsurance, and doughnut holes. Think, also, about how your prescription drug usage is trending. Are you using more drugs than last year? If so, you may use more yet next year. Don't assume that a current low level of drug use now will be predictive for your later years. Pick the one that works best for you, and decide if it's worth signing up for.

7. **Annual re-enrollment.** Once a year, you will be able to change to another Part D plan if you wish. Be sure to repeat steps 1 to 6 to evaluate what you should do.

If you don't take drugs, or you're currently spending less than the Medicare premium, you may conclude that Part D is not something that's worth your money. As long as you stay healthy, you are correct. But most people end up taking more and more drugs the older they get. Just remember that your insurance could cost you a lot more if you wait until you need the benefit. Signing up for a basic, low-cost Part D plan is a good idea even if you don't take any drugs currently.

ONCE YOU HAVE MEDICARE PART D DRUG COVERAGE, NOW WHAT?

It should be clear to you that getting Part D coverage is only half the battle. The average beneficiary can expect to save about 50% on his drugs by signing up for a Part D plan. The purpose of this book is to show you how to save another 50% or more on top of that. The techniques for doing this are the same as those detailed throughout the previous chapters. If you skipped them to read this chapter first, now is the time to go back and carefully read every chapter you missed (except for Chapter 10: "Free and Discounted Drug Programs," which is for non-Medicare consumers). Each of these chapters contains valuable information on how you can save hundreds or thousands of dollars a year on your Part D costs for your deductible, coinsurance, and the dread doughnut hole.

Know the System (Chapter 2). Understand the games the drugmakers play to get you to take the most expensive drugs. Know the system to beat the system.

Know the 7 Questions to Ask Your Doctor and Pharmacist (Chapter 4). Tell your doctor and your pharmacist you have to pay a big portion of your drug costs. Ask for their help. Ask them the seven key questions to make sure you always get the drugs you need at the lowest possible cost.

Know About OTC Medications and Dietary Supplements (Chapters 5 and 6). Find out about the thousands of inexpensive drugs you can buy over the counter, many of which were once available by prescription only. Learn how you can find what you need for a fraction of the cost of prescription drugs.

Know About Generic and Lower Cost Brand Name Drugs (Chapter 7). Learn why generic drugs are the best bargain in health care. If there are no generics for your condition, you may find

that your doctor has a wide choice of equally
effective brand name medications to prescribe
for you, some of which cost much less than
others.

Learn About Tablet Splitting (Chapter 8).
Learn how you can save up to 50% on your
drugs with this safe, proven technique that
has been used by doctors and their patients for
years.

**Know About the Double-Edged Sword of Free
Drug Samples (Chapter 9).** Learn how to tell the
difference between free samples that will save you
a lot of money and those that will actually
increase your costs.

**Know How to Be a Savvy Drug Shopper
(Chapter 11).** Once you have the prescription for
the right drug, use these techniques to find the
pharmacy that will provide it for you at the
lowest cost.

**Know About Your Importing Options (Chapter
12.)** Medicare Part D will not cover Canadian
drugs. However, you may find it useful to know
your options for buying lower cost imported
drugs, and whether you may be able to save
money this way.

Just remember, the new Medicare drug coverage
will not absolve you of the responsibility to work with
your doctors and pharmacists to get the drugs you
need at the lowest possible cost. The principles in this
book will help you do that. Good hunting.

APPENDICES

APPENDICES

APPENDIX A

7 QUESTIONS FOR YOUR DOCTOR AND WORKSHEET

DOCTOR, CAN I SAVE MONEY WITH:
1. Alternatives to drugs?
2. OTC drugs instead of Rx?
3. Generic drugs?
4. Lower-priced brand name drugs?
5. Tablet-splitting doses?
6. 100-day mail order Rx's?
7. Extra free samples?

7 Questions Worksheet

Complete and take with you to your doctor

List your Current Medications:	1. Alternatives to Meds?	2. OTC Alternatives?	3. Generic Alternatives?	4. Lower Cost Brand?	5. Tablet-Split Dose?	6. 100-Day Mail Order Rx?	7. Extra Free Samples
1.							
2.							
3.							
4.							
5.							
6.							
7.							
8.							

APPENDIX B

WORKSHEET: FIND THE RIGHT PRESCRIPTION DRUG DISCOUNT CARD

(See Chapter 10 for discussion on finding the right discount card.)

Drug, Form, Dose	Quantity	Price w/Card 1:	Price w/Card 2:	Price w/Card 3:	Price w/Card 4:
1.		$	$	$	$
2.		$	$	$	$
3.		$	$	$	$
4.		$	$	$	$
5.		$	$	$	$
6.		$	$	$	$
7.		$	$	$	$
8.		$	$	$	$
9.		$	$	$	$
10.		$	$	$	$
Drug Card Cost		$	$	$	$
Total Cost		$	$	$	$

APPENDIX C

ONLINE PHARMACY WEBSITES

If you want to buy your drugs online, or if you just want to check prices, here are some online pharmacy sites that I have found to be useful and reliable. This is hardly an exhaustive catalog, so feel free to use your own judgment and experience to expand your list.

Costco

(www.costco.com) Once on this site, click the "Pharmacy" link. It has some of the best retail prescription and OTC prices on the Web, especially for generic drugs, and you don't have to be a Costco member to purchase prescription drugs online.

Destination Rx

(www.destinationrx.com/default nonmember.asp) I really like this site. You enter a drug name, pick the dosage and quantity, and it will display retail prices from multiple online pharmacies, such as Costco, Walgreens, drugstore.com, AARP, and others.

Hyde Rx

(www.HydeRx.com) I maintain this site. I link it to various online pharmacies that I consider to offer low-cost, reliable, safe, fast service. I have no ownership interest in any pharmacy, and focus on finding the lowest prices available on the market. These links change from time to time.

Drugstore.com

(www.drugstore.com) The Internet bubble in the late 1990s and early 2000s spawned legions of online pharmacies that were going to revolutionize prescription drug retailing. Most of them are gone. Drugstore.com is one of the few survivors of the bubble burst, and I have had good experience buying their products.

Walgreens

(www.walgreens.com) This is a well-designed site with tons of useful information, including prescription drug prices. What makes this site unique is that you can order a drug online either to be shipped to your home or that you can pick up at one of their more than 4,000 retail stores. This is particularly handy if you find they have the lowest price for a drug you need right away, such as a pain medication or antibiotic.

Sam's Club and Wal-Mart

(www.samsclub.com and www.walmart.com) The Sam's Club site lets you look up drug prices and order refills to be picked up at a Sam's Club store. The Wal-Mart site also allows you to order refills for local pickup, but does not furnish prices online; you have to call the store for that.

Hillhurst Clinical Pharmacy

(**www.gracemeds.com**) This is a Canadian online pharmacy, located in Calgary, Alberta, that I have found to be reliable.

APPENDIX D

ONLINE DRUG INFORMATION

A good way to find out about a specific drug is to go to the Internet and enter the drug's name on a search engine, such as www.google.com, www.teoma.com, or www.yahoo.com. That's when the fun begins, as you face sorting through the several *hundred thousand* results that show up on your screen, ten at a time. Amidst the plethora of sites are many that are actually helpful, definitive, and not trying to sell you something—at least not directly. Others are hosted by the usual array of quacks, malcontents, and scam artists. Below are a few of the many sites that I have found to be reliable. If you see the following URL components in a search result, you're likely to get good information. You can also access these and other sites through my website at **www.HydeRx.com.** There are many, many more reliable sites than these few, so don't be afraid to use your judgment about gauging the veracity of other sites. Just be wary.

FDA-APPROVED PRESCRIPTION AND OTC DRUGS:

Medline

(www.nlm.nih.gov/medlineplus/) This site is maintained by the U.S. National Library of Medicine and the National Institutes of Health. It's definitive and is written in consumer-friendly language.

Drugs.com

(www.drugs.com) This site bills itself as "the most popular, comprehensive and up-to-date drug information resource online. Fast, easy searching of over 24,000 approved medications." "The Drugs.com drug-information database is powered by three independent leading medical-information suppliers: Physicians' Desk Reference, Cerner Multum, and Thomson Micromedex. Individual drug (or drug-class) information content compiled by these sources is delivered complete and unaltered by Drugs.com." The site is advertising supported, but does not directly sell drugs, nor is it affiliated with any drug company. In fact, it's owned by a couple of New Zealand pharmacists. Good site.

MedicineNet.com

(www.medicinenet.com) MedicineNet.com is an online, healthcare media publishing company. Another advertising-supported site, this one is produced by "a network of over 70 U.S. Board Certified Physicians" who also author *Webster's New World Medical Dictionary*.

Oddly, it was easier for me to find drug information on the site by using a search engine, such as google.com, teoma.com, or yahoo.com, to get directly to what I wanted than by trying to navigate this website itself. Good information, though.

RxList

(rxlist.com) Another advertising supported site, RxList does not sell drugs directly, but does refer you to an affiliated online pharmacy. This is another site that is easier to search from a search engine like Google, Teoma, or Yahoo! than from the site itself. While not as comprehensive as the above sites, the information seems pretty good.

Yahoo!Health

(http://health.yahoo.com/drug) Operated by the search engine company Yahoo!, this advertising supported site provides information produced by Healthwise, Incorporated, a not-for-profit organization long known for providing useful consumer healthcare information.

FDA Electronic Orange Book

(http://www.fda.gov/cder/ob/default.htm) This is the so-called FDA Electronic Orange Book. If you want to find out if a brand name drug is also available generically, this is a good site. It's operated by the FDA, and includes just about everything they've approved.

PDR*health*

(www.pdrhealth.com) PDR*health* is a consumer-friendly guide to prescription drugs, OTC medications, herbal medicines, and nutritional supplements. Doctors use the professional version of the PDR (Physician's Desk Reference) daily to review drugs before prescribing for their patients. This website is produced by the same folks, but in patient-friendly layman's language.

Center for Evidence Based Policy

(www.ohsu.edu/policycenter/) If you want to see head-to-head comparisons of different drugs in similar classes, this is *the* site for you. Heavy on technical and statistical language, it may not be for the casual laymen, but it provides an absolute wealth of information. Operated by the Center for Evidence Based Policy at the Oregon Health & Science University, this website shows the results of their exhaustive analyses of available clinical data on more than twenty different classes of drugs. It's too bad they don't go a step further to include actual drug costs and cost benefit analyses, but my hat's off to these people for a fine job. Presented in a more consumer-friendly format, their data could foster a revolution in cost-effective drug buying.

ClinicalTrials.gov

(www.clinicaltrials.gov/) Find a clinical trial on this government website by searching an extensive database of programs for which volunteers are being sought. The site provides an interactive search box into which you can enter one or more key words (e.g., "heart attack, Los Angeles"), and you will be able to browse all the various registered programs that fit your criteria. Just click on any program that looks interesting. I warn you that the language tends to be technical, but you may find something that looks interesting. If you do, you can contact the program via the contact information provided in the project description.

DIETARY SUPPLEMENTS:

M. D. Anderson

(http://www.mdanderson.org/departments/cimer/din dex.cfm?pn=6eb86a59-ebd9-11d4-810100508b603a14) Entering this terribly complicated Web address in your browser will ironically yield one of the more accessible and comprehensive sources of current information on a wide range of alternative, complementary, and integrative therapies (you can also just enter **www.mdander son.org,** but you'll have to do some further navigation once you're there). The website is maintained by the prestigious University of Texas M. D. Anderson Cancer Center and covers many therapies other than just cancer-related ones.

Memorial Sloan-Kettering Cancer Center

(http://www.mskcc.org/mskcc/html/11570.cfm) An encyclopedic, but rather technical site from Memorial Sloan-Kettering Cancer Center with information on many alternative therapies.

National Center for Complementary and Alternative Medicine

(http://nccam.nih.gov/clinicaltrials/treatment therapy.htm) If you're interested in participating in a clinical trial of alternative therapies, or if you just want to know the current state of scientific research, this website by the National Institutes of Health's National Center for Complementary and Alternative Medicine lists more than eighty trials currently recruiting patients or under way.

MedlinePlus

(http://www.nlm.nih.gov/medlineplus/comple mentaryandalternativetherapies.html) A service of the U.S. National Library of Medicine and the National Institutes of Health, MedlinePlus is a useful clearinghouse for information on dietary supplements and herbal treatments for different medical conditions.

Quackwatch

(www.quackwatch.org) This site administers a strong dose of sunlight to many of the darker corners of alternative therapy. It is maintained by Stephen Barrett, MD, a retired psychiatrist, and makes for fascinating reading.

APPENDIX E

OTC, GENERIC, AND BRAND NAME ALTERNATIVES BY THERAPEUTIC CATEGORY

(Note: Brand name drugs are capitalized; generic drugs are lowercase.)

Allergy, Cough & Cold		
Brand Rx		
Allegra	Beconase AQ	Nasonex
Allegra-D	Flonase	Rhinocort Aqua
Astelin	Nasacort AQ	Zyrtec

Allergy, Cough & Cold (cont'd)

OTC Generic (Brand)

chlorpheniramine (Chlor-Trimeton)	guaifenesin (Robitussin)	phenylephrine (Neo-Synephrine)
clemastine (Tavist)	loratadine (Claritin)	phenylpropanola-mine
dextromethorphan (Robitussin DM)	oxymetazoline (Afrin)	pseudoephedrine (Sudafed)
diphenhydramine (Benadryl)		

Generic Rx

chlorpheniramine	diphenhydramine	hydroxyzine*
cyproheptadine	fexofenadine and pseudoephedrine (Allegra-D)	promethazine
dexchlorpheniramine	guaifenesin/codeine	

*Ask your doctor or pharmacist about tablet splitting.

Anti-Spasticity and Muscle Relaxants		
Brand Rx		
Dantrium	Zanaflex	

OTC Generic (Brand)		
methocarbamol (Robaxacet [OTC in Canada only])		

Generic Rx		
baclofen	carisoprodol	cyclobenzaprine* (Flexeril)

*Ask your doctor or pharmacist about tablet splitting.

Asthma and Obstructive Pulmonary Disease		
Brand Rx		
Accolate*	Flovent	Serevent
Advair Diskus	Foradil	Singulair*
Alupent	Proventil HFA	Theo-24
Azmacort	Pulmicort	Uniphyl
Combivent	Qvar	

OTC Generic (Brand)		
ephedrine	epinephrine	

Generic Rx		
albuterol (Proventil)	isoproterenol	terbutaline
ipratropium (Atrovent) isoproterenol	metaproterenol (Proventil)	theophylline

*Ask your doctor or pharmacist about tablet splitting.

Blood Pressure/Angina/Cardiac/Thrombosis

Brand Rx

Aceon*	Demadex	Mavik
Aggrenox	Diovan	Monopril*
Agrylin	Diovan HCT*	Nimotop
Atacand*	DynaCirc CR	Norvasc*
Adalat CC	Flomax	Plavix*
Altace	Innohep	Plendil
Avapro*	Lanoxin*	Toprol XL*
Catapres TTS	Lotensin	Tracleer
Coreg*	Lotensin HCT	Univasc*
Cozaar	Lotrel	Verelan PM
Coumadin*	Lovenox	

OTC Generic (Brand)

N/A		

*Ask your doctor or pharmacist about tablet splitting.

Blood Pressure/Angina/Cardiac/Thrombosis (cont'd)		
Generic Rx		
acebutolol	doxazosin* (Cardura)	lisinopril* (Prinivil, Zestril)
amiloride and HCTZ	enalapril* (Vasotec)	lisinopril HCTZ
atenolol	furosemide* (Lasix)	metoprolol* (Toprol)
atenolol and chlorthalidone	guanabenz	nadolol* (Corgard)
bisoprolol/HCTZ	HCTZ/triamterene*	propranolol* (Inderal)
bumetanide	HCTZ/spironolactone	quinapril (Accupril)*
captopril* (Capoten)	hydralazine	quinapril HCTZ (Accuretic)
chlorthalidone	hydrochlorothiazide*	spironolactone* (Aldactone)
clonidine* (Catapres)	indapamide	verapamil* (Verelan)
diltiazem* (Cardizem SR and CD)	labetalol* (Normodyne)	warfarin (Coumadin)

*Ask your doctor or pharmacist about tablet splitting.

Cancer and Immunosuppression Drugs		
Brand Rx		
Alkeran	Estinyl	Matulane
Ceenu	Fluoroplex	Nolvadex
Efudex	Gleevec	

OTC Generic (Brand)		
N/A		

Generic Rx		
cyclosporine	fluorouracil	tamoxifen
diethylstilbestrol	megestrol	

*Ask your doctor or pharmacist about tablet splitting.

Cholesterol Reduction		
Brand Rx		
Advicor	Lescol XL	Zetia
Colestid	Lipitor*	Zocor*
Crestor	Pravachol*	
Lescol	Tricor	

OTC Generic (Brand)		
red rice yeast	oat bran	psyllium fiber (Metamucil)

Generic Rx		
cholestyramine	gemfibrozil* (Lopid)	niacin
clofibrate	lovastatin* (Mevacor)	

*Ask your doctor or pharmacist about tablet splitting.

Contraceptives—Oral		
Brand Rx		
Estrostep FE	Nor-QD	Trivora
Loestrin	Plan B	Yasmin
Loestrin Fe	Tri-Norinyl	

OTC Generic (Brand)		
N/A		

Generic Rx		
Genora	N.E.E.	Norehin
Necon	Nelova	

*Ask your doctor or pharmacist about tablet splitting.

Depression/Anxiety/Bipolar/OCD		
Brand Rx		
Effexor* Effexor XR	Eskalith CR Lexapro	Wellbutrin SR Zoloft*

OTC Generic (Brand)		
Saint-John's-Wort		

Generic Rx		
alprazolam* (Xanax)	desipramine (Norpramin)	nefazodone (Serzone)
amitriptyline	doxepin	nortriptyline
amoxapine	fluoxetine* (Prozac)	paroxetine (Paxil)
bupropion (Wellbutrin)	fluvoxamine (Luvox)	protriptyline
buspirone* (BuSpar)	imipramine	trazodone* (Desyrel)
citalopram* (Celexa)	mirtazapine (Remeron)	
clomipramine		

*Ask your doctor or pharmacist about tablet splitting.

Diabetes		
Brand Rx		
Actos*	Glucovance	Novolog
Amaryl*	Humalog	Prandin
Avandia*	Humulin	Precose
Glucagon	Lantus	Starlix
Glucotrol XL	Novolin	

OTC Generic (Brand)		
N/A		

Generic Rx		
chlorpropamide	glyburide* (DiaBeta)	tolbutamide
glipizide* (Glucotrol)	metformin* (Glucophage)	

*Ask your doctor or pharmacist about tablet splitting.

Erectile Dysfunction		
Brand Rx		
Cialis	Levitra*	Viagra*

OTC Generic (Brand)		
N/A		

Generic Rx		
N/A		

GI Drugs—Other		
Brand Rx		
Asacol	Cytotec	Rowasa
Canasa	Golytely	URSO
Colazal	Lotronex*	Zelnorm*
Colyte	Pancrease MT	
Creon	Pentasa	

*Ask your doctor or pharmacist about tablet splitting.

GI Drugs—Other (cont'd)

OTC Generic (Brand)

N/A		

Generic Rx

dicyclomine	hyoscyamine	pancrelipase
hydrocortisone rectal	hyoscyamine/atrop/scop	propantheline
	lactulose	sulfasalazine

Heart Rhythm and Cardiac Vasodilators

Brand Rx

Deponit	Nitrolingual Pumpspray	Tambocor
Nitro-Dur	Nitrostat	Tonocard
Nitrol	Norpace CR	

*Ask your doctor or pharmacist about tablet splitting.

Heart Rhythm and Cardiac Vasodilators (cont'd)		
OTC Generic (Brand)		
N/A		

Generic Rx		
amiodarone	isoxsuprine	propafenone
digoxin and digitoxin	mexiletine	quinidine gluconate
disopyramide	nitroglycerin SL topical	quinidine sulfate
isosorbide dinitrate	procainamide	

Heartburn and GI Acid Suppression		
Brand Rx		
AcipHex	Prevacid	Protonix
Nexium	Prevpac	

*Ask your doctor or pharmacist about tablet splitting.

Heartburn and GI Acid Suppression (cont'd)		
OTC Generic (Brand)		
cimetidine (Tagamet)	nizatidine (Axid) omeprazole (Prilosec OTC)	ranitidine (Zantac)

Generic Rx		
cimetidine (Tagamet) famotidine* (Pepcid)	metoclopramide* (Reglan) nizatidine (Axid)	ranitidine* (Zantac) sucralfate

Hormone Replacement		
Brand Rx		
Activella	Estratest H.S.	Premphase
Alora	Estring	Prempro
Aygestin	Evista	Testaderm TTS
Climara	Femhrt	Vagifem
Combipatch	Ortho-Prefest	Vivelle
Estratest	Premarin*	

*Ask your doctor or pharmacist about tablet splitting.

Hormone Replacement (cont'd)		
OTC Generic (Brand)		
N/A		

Generic Rx		
estradiol estropipate* (Ortho-EST)	generic Estraderm generic Estratab	medroxyprogesterone

Infection—Bacterial		
Brand Rx		
Biaxin XL	Levaquin*	Suprax
Ceftin	Mepron	Tequin
Cefzil	Omnicef	Vantin
Cipro	Primsol	Zithromax
Duricef	Rifamate	Zyvox

*Ask your doctor or pharmacist about tablet splitting.

Infection—Bacterial (cont'd)		
OTC Generic (Brand)		
bacitracin (Baciguent) bacitracin zinc bacitracin zinc-neomycin-polymyxin B (Neomixin, Neosporin Original)	bacitracin zinc–polymyxin B ointment, aerosol, or powder (Polysporin, Polysporin Powder) chlortetracycline	hydrochloride (Achromycin) hydrochloride (Aureomycin) neomycin neomycin sulfate tetracycline

Generic Rx		
amoxicillin (Amoxil) amoxicillin and clavulanate* (Augmentin) ampicillin cefadroxil cephalexin* cephradine	clindamycin dicloxacillin doxycycline* erythromycin metronidazole* (Flagyl)	minocycline nitrofurantoin penicillin VK* SMX/TMP (generic Septra) tetracycline

*Ask your doctor or pharmacist about tablet splitting.

Infection—Fungal		
Brand Rx		
Diflucan	Lamisil	Vfend

OTC (topical only) Generic (Brand)		
clioquinol (Vioform) clotrimazole (Lotrimin, Mycelex)	miconazole (Monistat, Absorbine, Athlete's Foot,Breezee Mist, Fungoid Crème, Lotrimin AF powder)	tolnaftate (Aftate, Tinactin, Ting) undecylenic acid (Cruex, Desenex)

Generic Rx		
generic Fulvicin P/G	generic Mycostatin	generic Nizoral

*Ask your doctor or pharmacist about tablet splitting.

Infection—Viral		
Brand Rx		
Combivir	Norvir	Valtrex*
Cytovene	Rebetron	Videx
Epivir	Retrovir	Viracept
Famvir	Tamiflu	
Flumadine	Valcyte	

OTC Generic (Brand)		
N/A		

Generic Rx		
acyclovir (Zovirax)*	amantadine	rimantadine

Insomnia—Sleep Agents		
Brand Rx		
Ambien*	Sonata	

*Ask your doctor or pharmacist about tablet splitting.

Insomnia—Sleep Agents (cont'd)		
OTC Generic (Brand)		
diphenhydramine (Benadryl, Compoz, Nytol, Sominex)	doxylamine succinate (Unisom Sleep Tabs)	

Generic Rx		
estazolam	lorazepam* (Ativan)	triazolam
flurazepam	temazepam	

Muscle Relaxants and Other Drugs		
Brand Rx		
Actonel	Detrol	Intron A
Androderm	Ditropan XL	Miacalcin
Androgel	Epogen	Neulasta
Aranesp	Evoxac	Neupogen
Aricept*	Gonal-F	Orapred
Cetrotide	Humegon	PEG-Intron

*Ask your doctor or pharmacist about tablet splitting.

Muscle Relaxants and Other Drugs (cont'd)		
Brand Rx		
Procrit Repronex	Skelaxin* Synarel	Xenical Xyrem

OTC Generic (Brand)		
Robaxin (Canada only as OTC)		

Generic Rx		
clomiphene leuprolide	nicotine transdermal oxybutynin	pentoxifylline ticlodipine

Pain—Joint Inflammation and Headache		
Brand Rx		
Arava Arthrotec	Bextra Celebrex*	Enbrel Kineret

*Ask your doctor or pharmacist about tablet splitting.

Pain—Joint Inflammation and Headache (cont'd)

OTC Generic (Brand)		
acetaminophen (Tylenol)	aspirin (Ascriptin, Bayer, Bufferin, Ecotrin)	ibuprofen (Advil, Motrin) naproxen (Aleve)

Generic Rx		
diclofenac (Cataflam)	ketoprofen	naproxen (Naprosyn)
etodolac (Lodine)	ketorolac	naproxen sodium*
ibuprofen* (Advil, Nuprin, Motrin)	methylprenisolone* (Medrol)	oxaprozin
		piroxicam
indomethacin	nabumetone	salsalate
		sulindac

*Ask your doctor or pharmacist about tablet splitting.

Pain—Migraine Syndrome		
Brand Rx		
Amerge Imitrex	Maxalt Migranal	Relpax Zomig

OTC Generic (Brand)		
acetaminophen (Tylenol)	aspirin (Ascriptin, Bayer, Bufferin, Ecotrin)	ibuprofen (Advil, Motrin) caffeine

Generic Rx		
APAP combinations ASA combinations	beta-blockers (e.g. atenolol*) calcium blockers (verapamil)	tricyclics (e.g. amitriptyline*)

*Ask your doctor or pharmacist about tablet splitting.

Pain—Oral Analgesics

Brand Rx

Actiq	MS Contin	OxyContin
Duragesic	MSIR	

OTC Generic (Brand)

acetaminophen (Tylenol)	ibuprofen (Advil, Motrin)	naproxen (Aleve)
aspirin (Ascriptin, Bayer, Bufferin, Ecotrin)	ketoprofen (Orudis KT)	

Generic Rx

APAP/narcotic combinations* (Vicodin, Percocet)	meperidine	propoxyphene and acetaminophen* (Darvocet)
ASA/narcotic combinations	oxycodone	tramadol* (Ultram)
	propoxyphene	

*Ask your doctor or pharmacist about tablet splitting.

Parkinson's Disease and Multiple Sclerosis

Brand Rx

Avonex	Copaxone	Rebif
Betaseron	Mirapex	ReQuip
Comptan	Permax	

OTC Generic (Brand)

N/A		

Generic Rx

amantadine	bromocriptine	selegiline
benztropine	carbidopa-levodopa CR	trihexyphenidyl
biperiden		

Psychoses

Brand Rx

Risperdal*	Seroquel*	Zyprexa*

*Ask your doctor or pharmacist about tablet splitting.

Psychoses (cont'd)		
OTC Generic (Brand)		
N/A		

Generic Rx		
chlorpromazine	loxapine	thiothixene
fluphenazine	perphenazine	trifluoperazine
haloperidol	thioridazine	

Seizures & Convulsions		
Brand Rx		
Depakote	Gabitril	Topamax*
Depakote ER	Keppra	Trileptal
Dilantin	Tegretol XR	Zonegran

*Ask your doctor or pharmacist about tablet splitting.

Seizures & Convulsions (cont'd)		
OTC Generic (Brand)		
N/A		

Generic Rx		
carbamazepine	diazepam* (Valium)	phenytoin
clonazepam* (Klonopin)	gabapentin (Neurontin)	primidone
clorazepate	phenobarbital	valproic acid

Stimulants—Narcolepsy & ADHD Only		
Brand Rx		
Adderall XR	Metadate ER	Ritalin-LA
Metadate CD	Provigil	Strattera

*Ask your doctor or pharmacist about tablet splitting.

Stimulants—Narcolepsy & ADHD Only (cont'd)		
OTC Generic (Brand)		
N/A		

Generic Rx		
dextroamphetamine	methylphenidate & SR	pemoline

Thyroid		
OTC Generic (Brand)		
N/A		

Generic Rx		
levothyroxine* (Levothroid, Levoxyl, Synthroid*)		

*Ask your doctor or pharmacist about tablet splitting.

Topicals—Infection and Acne

Brand Rx

BenzaClin	MetroCream	Retin-A Micro
Differin	MetroGel	Spectazole
Loprox	Oxistat	Tazorac

OTC Generic (Brand)

bacitracin (Baciguent)	polymyxin B (Neomixin, Neosporin Original)	miconazole (Monistat, Absorbine Athlete's Foot, Breezee Mist, Fungoid Crème, Lotrimin AF powder)
bacitracin zinc		
chlortetracycline hydrochloride (Aureomycin)	bacitracin zinc-polymyxin B ointment, aerosol or powder (Polysporin, Polysporin Powder)	
neomycin sulfate (Neomycin, Myciguent Cream)		undecylenic acid (Cruex, Desenex)
tetracycline hydrochloride (Achromycin)	tolnftate (Aftate, Tinactin, Ting)	clioquinol (Vioform)
bacitracin zinc-neomycin-	clotrimazole (Lotrimin, Mycelex)	benzoyl peroxide (Clearasil, Oxy 10)

*Ask your doctor or pharmacist about tablet splitting.

Topicals—Infection and Acne (cont'd)		
Generic Rx		
clindamycin generic Accutane generic Mycolog II	generic Retin-A gentamicin erythromycin	ketoconazole silver sulfadiazine

Topicals—Infection—GYN		
Brand Rx		
Cleocin Cleocin T	MetroGel	Terazol

OTC Generic (Brand)		

butoconazole nitrate
  (Femstat 3)
 	
clotrimazole
  (Gyne-Lotrimin)
	miconazole
	  (Monistat 7)*
		tioconazole
		  (Vagistat 1)

*Ask your doctor or pharmacist about tablet splitting.

Topicals—Infection—GYN (cont'd)		
Generic Rx		
nystatin vaginal	triple sulfa vaginal	

Topicals—Inflammation		
Brand Rx		
Aclovate	Elidel	Regranex
Diprolene	Elocon	Soriatane
Diprolene AF	Protopic	Ultravate

OTC Generic (Brand)		
benzocaine (Bactine, Lanacane, Solarcaine)	hydrocortisone (Caldecort, Cortaid, Lanacort)	trolamine salicylate (Aspercreme, Sportscreme)
capsaicin	menthol, wintergreen oil, eucalyptus oil (BenGay, Icy Hot)	zinc (calamine)
dibucaine (Nupercainal)		

*Ask your doctor or pharmacist about tablet splitting.

Topicals—Inflammation (cont'd)

Generic Rx

betamethasone	desoximetasone	fluocinonide
clobetasol	diflorasone	hydrocortisone valerate
desonide	fluocinolone	triamcinolone

Topicals—Eye

Brand Rx

Alphagan-P	Lumigan	Voltaren Ophth
Alomide	Ocuflox	Xalatan
Azopt	Patanol	Zaditor
Livostin	Tobradex	

OTC Generic (Brand)

antazoline phosphate & naphazoline hydrochloride (Vasocon-A)	glycerin, hypromellose, & polyethylene glycol (Visine Tears) naphazoline hydrochloride, &	pheniramine (Opcon-A, Visine-A) polyvinyl alcohol & povidone (Murine Tears)

*Ask your doctor or pharmacist about tablet splitting.

Topicals—Eye (cont'd)		
Generic Rx		
atropine	levobunolol	sulfacetamide-phenylephrine
bacitracin-neomycin-maleatepolymyxin B	naphazoline-antazoline	timolol gel
bacitracin-polymyxin B	neomycin-gramicidin-polymyxin B	tobramycin
carbachol	neomycin-dexamethasone	trimethoprim-polymyxin B (Polytrim)
dipivefrin	pilocarpine	trimethoprim and sulfamethoxazole* (Septra)
fluorometholone	prednisolone	
gentamicin sulfate	sulfacetamide-Prednisolone	

Topicals—Ear		
Brand Rx		
Cerumenex	Cortane-B	Floxin Otic

*Ask your doctor or pharmacist about tablet splitting.

Topicals—Ear (cont'd)		
OTC Generic (Brand)		
acetic acid and aluminum acetate (Star-Otic)	carbamide peroxide (Auro Ear Drops Debrox, E-R-O Drops, Murine Ear)	isopropyl alcohol (Auro-Dri, Swim Ear)

Generic Rx		
acetic acid-hydrocortisone	antipyrine-benzocaine	HC-neomycin-polymyxin B

Vertigo and Nausea		
Brand Rx		
Compazine	Torecan	Zofran

OTC Generic (Brand)		
cyclizine (Marezine)	dimenhydrinate (Dramamine)	ginger meclizine* (Bonine)

*Ask your doctor or pharmacist about tablet splitting.

Vertigo and Nausea (cont'd)		
Generic Rx		
prochlorperazine	promethazine* (Phenergan)	trimethobenzamide

*Ask your doctor or pharmacist about tablet splitting.

APPENDIX F

RECENT AND UPCOMING BRAND NAME DRUG PATENT EXPIRATIONS

(Note: The actual availability of generic drugs often lags behind the expiration date. You can find the latest generic status of any drug on the FDA's Electronic Orange Book website at http://www.fda.gov/cder/ob/default.htm.)

Brand Name (generic name)	Indication	Expiration	Patent Holder
Advair (fluticasone/ salmeterol)	Asthma	10/2008	GlaxoSmithKline
Allegra (fexofenadine)	Allergy	4/2005	Aventis
Altace (ramipril)	Hypertension	7/2005	King
Ambien (zolpidem)	Insomnia	4/2007	Sanofi
Axid (nizatidine)	Acid reflux, ulcer	4/2002	Reliant
Biaxin (clarithromycin)	Antibiotic	5/2005	Abbott
Cefzil (cefprozil)	Antibiotic	12/2005	BMS

Brand Name (generic name)	Indication	Expiration	Patent Holder
Celexa (citalopram)	Depression	7/2003	Forest
Cipro (ciprofloxacin)	Infection	2003	Bayer
Clarinex (desloratadine)	Allergy	1/2007	Schering-Plough
Claritin (loratadine)	Allergy	2002	Schering-Plough
Cytovene (ganciclovir)	CMV Virus	6/2003	Roche
Effexor XR (venlafaxine)	Depression	6/2008	Wyeth
Evista (raloxifene)	Osteoporosis	12/2002	Lilly
Flovent (fluticasone)	Asthma	11/2003	GlaxoSmithKline
Fosamax (alendronate)	Osteoporosis	2/2008	Merck
Glucophage XL (metformin)	Diabetes	10/2003	Bristol-Myers Squibb
Glucophage XR (metformin)	Diabetes	4/2006	Bristol-Myers Squibb
Imitrex (sumatriptan)	Migraine	6/2007	GlaxoSmithKline
Lamictal (lamotrigine)	Seizures, bipolar disorder	1/2009	GlaxoSmithKline

Brand Name (generic name)	Indication	Expiration	Patent Holder
Lexapro (escitalopram)	Depression	12/2009	Forest
Lipitor (atorvastatin)	Cholesterol	2010	Pfizer
Lotensin (benazepril)	Hypertension	8/2003	Novartis
Lovenox (enoxaparin)	Deep vein thrombosis	6/2005	Aventis
Mevacor (lovastatin)	Cholesterol	6/2001	Merck
Neurontin (gabapentin)	Epilepsy	2002	Pfizer
Norvasc (amlodipine)	Hypertension	1/2007	Pfizer
Paxil (paroxetine)	Depression	2006	GlaxoSmithKline
Pepcid (famotidine)	Acid reflux, ulcer	2000	Merck
Plavix (clopidogrel)	Thrombotic event risk	7/2003	Bristol-Myers Squibb
Pravachol (pravastatin)	Cholesterol	4/2006	Bristol-Myers Squibb
Prevacid (lansoprazole)	Acid reflux, ulcer	2005	Tap

Brand Name (generic name)	Indication	Expiration	Patent Holder
Prilosec (omeprazole)	Acid reflux, ulcer	2003	AstraZeneca
Prinivil	Hypertension	2001	Merck
Propecia (finasteride)	Hair growth	6/2006	Merck
Proscar (finasteride)	Benign prostatic hyperplasia	6/2006	Merck
Prozac (fluoxetine)	Depression	2/2001	Lilly
Requip (ropinirole)	Restless legs syndrome	12/2002	GlaxoSmithKline
Risperdal (risperidone)	Schizophrenia	6/2008	Janssen
Serzone (nefazodone)	Depression	3/2003	Bristol-Myers Squibb
Singulair (montelukast)	Asthma	2003	Merck
Sonata (zaleplon)	Insomnia	12/2008	Jones
Ultram (tramadol)	Pain	6/2003	Ortho-McNeil
Vasotec (enalpril)	Blood pressure	2003	Biovail
Wellbutrin (bupropion)	Depression	6/2004	GlaxoSmithKline

Brand Name (generic name)	Indication	Expiration	Patent Holder
Wellbutrin XL (bupropion)	Depression	8/2006	GlaxoSmithKline
Xalatan (latanoprost)	Glaucoma	1/2007	Pharmacies and Upjohn
Zestril (lisinopril)	Hypertension	2002	AstraZeneca
Zithromax (azithromycin)	Antibiotic	11/2005	Pfizer
Zocor (simvastatin)	Cholesterol	6/2006	Merck
Zofran (ondansetron)	Nausea	7/2005	GlaxoSmithKline
Zoloft (sertraline)	Depression	6/2006	Pfizer
Zyrtec (cetirizine)	Allergy	12/2007	Pfizer

APPENDIX G

NATIONAL, STATE, AND DRUG COMPANY ASSISTANCE PROGRAMS

When I began writing this book, I expected to have to research information on the several hundred drug assistance programs available throughout the United States. Fortunately, there is now a single free access point for almost all of these programs. It is called the Partnership for Prescription Assistance (PPA). PPA is a nonprofit partnership of drug companies, healthcare providers, patient advocates, and community groups that provides assistance to uninsured and low-income patients who may have difficulty paying for their medications. Through it, you can quickly—and at no charge—determine which programs are the most likely to offer what you need. Chapter 10 provides the details on how to access and use this program. Their website is at **www.pparx.org**.

NOTES

Chapter 1: Who Is This Book For? Everybody Who Uses Prescription Drugs

1 Seidman, Robert, Chief Pharm. Officer, WellPoint
2 Kalra, Ritu, "Health Benefit Bill Proceeds," *Hartford Courant*, 22 April 2005 [online]
3 "AHIP Finds More Than a Million Have HSAs," Benefit-News.com, accessed 5 May 2005
4 U.S. Depart of Labor, Bureau of Labor Statistics, available online at ftp://ftp.bls.gov/pub/special.requests/cpi/cpiai.txt

Chapter 2: Why Drugs Cost So Much: Know the System to Beat the System

1 Anand, Geeta, "Italian Drug Firm Draws Fire for Boosting Prices," *The Wall Street Journal*, June 2005, B5
2 Hensley, Scott, "As Drug-Sales Teams Multiply, Doctors Start to Tune Them Out," *The Wall Street Journal*, 13 June 2003 [online]
3 "Chapter 8: Health Care Costs, Pressure of Prescription Drug Costs," *Covering Health Issues, 2003, A Sourcebook for Journalists*, January 2003, available online at http://www.all-health.org/sourcebook2002/ch8_6.html
4 GenericSelect, "Blue Cross of California, Blue Cross Blue Shield of Georgia and Blue Cross Blue Shield of Missouri," *Blue Cross Blue Shield Association,* May 2004, available online at http://www.bcbs.com/blueworks/drugs/genericse lect.html
5 "Health Insurance Cost," National Coalition on Health Care, available online at http://www.nchc.org/facts/cost.shtml

6 O'Connell, Vanessa, "Drug Requests Are More Specific," *The Wall Street Journal,* 15 April 2002

7 Hensley, Scott, "Some Drug Makers Are Starting To Curtail TV Ad Spending," *The Wall Street Journal,* 16 May 2005, B1

8 Brownlee, Shannon and Jeanne Lenzer, "How Drug Companies Keep Tabs on Physicians," *Slate,* 31 May 2005 [online] http://slate.MSN.com/id/2119712/

9 Ibid

10 Hensley, "Drug-Sales Teams"

11 Tansey, Bernadette, "Why Doctors Prescribe Off Label," *San Francisco Chronicle,* 1 May 2005 available online at http://www.sfgate.com/cgi-bin/article.cgi?f=/c/a/2005/05/01/MNG10CI3M71.DTL

12 Carey, John and Amy Barrett, "'Off-Label'—And Out of Bounds?" *Business Week,* 18 October 2004, p. 39

13 Brownlee, "Keep Tabs"

14 Hensley, "Curtail"

15 O'Connell, "Drug Requests"

16 "Tufts Center for the Study of Drug Development Pegs Cost of a New Prescription Medicine at $802 Million," *Tufts Center for the Study of Drug Development,* 30 November 2001, available online at http://csdd.tufts.edu/NewsEvents/RecentNews.asp?newsid=6

17 Mullin, Rick, "Drug Development Costs About $1.7 Billion," *Chemical & Engineering News,* 15 December 2003 available online at http://pubs.acs.org/cen/topstory/8150/8150notw5.html

18 Carey, "Off-Label"

19 Rudavsky, Shari, "Parents Asked to Fight Overuse of Antibiotics," *The Boston Globe,* 7 October 2003

20 O'Neill, P, "Acute Otitis Media," *Clinical Evidence (7),* 236–242

21 De Ferranti, SD, et al, "Are Amoxicillin and Folate Inhibitors as Effective as Other Antibiotics for Acute Sinusitis? A Meta-Analysis." *BMJ,* 317(7159), 632–637

22 Hensley, "Curtail"

23 Hensley, Scott, "Ads Boost Consumer Awareness of Drugs,

but Downplay Risks," *The Wall Street Journal*, 31 March 2003

Chapter 4: Consult Your Biggest Allies: Seven Questions to Ask Your Doctor and Pharmacist

1 Gladwell, Malcolm, "High Prices," *The New Yorker*, 25 October 2004, available online at http://www.newyorker.com/critics/atlarge/?041025crat_atlarge
2 Vesely, Rebecca, "Kaiser Halts Doctors' Freebies," *Inside Bay Area*, date unknown, available online at http://www.insidebayarea.com/portlet/article/html/fragments/print_article.jsp?article=2681048
3 Robeznieks, Andis, "Doctors Mindful of Patients' Out-of-Pocket Drug Costs," *AMNews*, 2 May 2005

Chapter 5: What About Over-the-Counter Drugs?

1 Strom, Brian L, "Statins and Over-the-Counter Availability," *The New England Journal of Medicine*, 7 April 2005, 1403–1405
2 Schmid, Randolph E, "Non-Prescription Drugs a Mixed Bag," *Seattle Post-Intelligencer*, 29 August 2002
3 "Diphenhydramine Oral," *National Library of Medicine Medlineplus*, accessed 27 June 2005, available online at http://www.nlm.nih.gov/medlineplus/druginfo/medmaster/a682539.html.
4 Horstman, Barry M, "George Rieveschl: Sneezers Can Thank Him for Relief," *Cincinnati Post*, 1 November 1999
5 Snowbeck, Christopher, "FDA Raises Hurdle for Drugs to Move From Prescription To Over-the-Counter," *Pittsburgh Post-Gazette*, 16 January 2005
6 Strom, "Statins"
7 Schmit, Julie, "Switching to Aspirin for Pain Relief? Beware Its Risks, Too," *USA Today*, 13 January 2005, available online at http://www.usatoday.com/news/health/2005-01-13-aspirin_x.htm

8 Strom, "Statins"

9 Pressler, Margaret Webb, "Retailers Restrict Some Cold Medicines," *Washington Post*, 14 May 2005, A01

10 "A Victory for Women," *New York Times*, 24 June 2005

11 Schmid, "Mixed Bag"

12 "FDA Set to Decide on Morning-After Pill," *The Associated Press*, 17 January 2005

13 Harris, Gardiner, "Schering-Plough Faces a Future With Coffers Unfortified by Claritin," *The Wall Street Journal*, 22 March 2002

14 Ibid

15 "Claritin Allergy 24-Hour" (advertisement), *Colorado Springs Gazette*, 15 December 2002

Chapter 6: What About Dietary Supplements and Herbal Medications?

1 Landro, Laura, "Where to Find Reliable Sources on Alternative Medicine," *The Wall Street Journal*, 21 October 2003

2 Marx, Bonnie, "Complementary and Alternative Medicines: What Our Doctors Need to Know," *Southern Illinois University Focal Point*, February 2001, available online at http://news.siu.edu/focalpoint/feb2001/story5.html

3 "Herbal Supplements," *Mayo Clinic*, 2004

4 Marks, "Complementary"

5 "FDA Approves Sale of Prescription Placebo," *The Onion*, accessed 18 September 2003, available online at http://www.the-onion.com/3936/news2.html

6 "All in the mind," *The Economist*, 11 March 2002, 83

Chapter 7: Go Generic or Switch to Lower-Priced Brands

1 "About Generic Pharmaceuticals," *The National Association of Chain Drug Stores* accessed 1 June 2005, available online at http://www.gphaonline.org/aboutgenerics/index.html

2 "FDA Ensures Equivalence of Generic Drugs," *FDA Center for Drug Evaluation and Research Special Report*, August 2002, available online at www.fda.gov/cder

3 Nightingale, Stuart L. "Therapeutic Equivalence of Generic Drugs Letter to Health Practitioners," 28 January 1998, available online at www.fda.gov/cder/news/nightgenlett.htm

4 "FDA Ensures"

5 Nightingale, "Therapeutic"

6 Ibid

7 Angell, Marcia. *The Truth About Drug Companies: How They Deceive Us and What to Do About It.* (New York: Random House)

8 "Pfizer Is Urged to Split Its Cholesterol Drugs," *Los Angeles Times (Bloomberg News)*, accessed June 2005, available online from http://www.latimes.com/business/la-fi-pfizer23jun23, 1,7791877.story

Chapter 8: Split Your Pills—and Costs—in Half

1 Cross, Margaret Ann, "Two for the Price of One: Beauty of Pill-Splitting Catches On," *Managed Care Magazine*, accessed 27 August 2005, available online at http://www.managedcaremag.com/archives/0302/0302.pillsplitting.html

Chapter 10: Free and Discounted Drug Programs

1 "PowerPoint Presentation at Harvard Business School Alumni Health Care Conference," *Blue Cross Blue Shield*, December 2003

2 Lueck, Sarah, "In Mississippi, Governor Sees 'Cancer on Our Finances' Amid $268 Million Gap—New Pressure From Bush Cuts," *The Wall Street Journal*, 7 February 2005, A1

3 "Medicaid: A Brief Summary," *Centers for Medicare & Medicaid Services (CMS)*, 3 December 2004, available online at http://www.cms.hhs.gov/publications/overview-medicare-medicaid/default4.asp

4 "What Is the Partnership for Prescription Assistance?"

[online] accessed 15 May 2005, available online at https://www.pparx.org/Intro.php

5 Snyder, Jodie, "Grocers Offering Prescription Discounts to Woo Uninsured," *The Arizona Republic*, 21 June 2005

6 Bureau of Primary Health Care "Program Information," accessed 1 June 2005, available online at http://bphc.hrsa.gov/programs/CHCPrograminfo.asp

Chapter 11: Savvy Shopping: Getting the Best Deal from Retail, Mail Order, and Internet Pharmacies

1 Caffrey, Andrew and Russell Gold, "States Find Big Variations in Drug Prices," *The Wall Street Journal*, 6 March 2002

2 Martinez, Barbara, "Generic Drugs By Mail Can Be a Raw Deal," *The Wall Street Journal*, 15 February 2005, B1

3 Meyer, Paul, "McKinney, Texas, Drugstore Offers Prescriptions at No Profit for Needy," *The Dallas Morning News*, 20 August 2004, available online at http://www.pnhp.org/news/2004/august/mckinney_texas_drugs.php

4 Querna, Elizabeth, "Prices at Nearby Drugstores Vary by Huge Amounts," *US News & World Report*, 20 September 2004, available online at http://www.usnews.com/usnews/health/articles/040920/20drugstore.htm

5 Ibid

6 "Rx Report Shows Drug Prices Rose 7.1% in 2004," *BenefitNews.com*, accessed 12 April 2005

7 "Producer Prices Jumped Last Month, Rising 0.6%," *The Wall Street Journal*, 17 May 2005

8 Schultz, Marisa, "Pharmacy Mistakes Kill, Injure Thousands," *The Detroit News*, 14 April 2003

9 Ruethling, Gretchen, "Almost All Libraries Offer Free Web Access," *New York Times*, 24 June 2005

Chapter 12: Oh, Canada!

1 Harris, Gardiner, "Drug Makers' New Intensity in Defense of U.S. Borders," *New York Times*, 30 October 2003

2 Horowitz, David J, "Letter," *FDA*, accessed 30 June 2003,

available online at http://www.fda.gov/foi/warning_letters/
g4376d.htm

3 "Canada Plans to Restrict Internet Drug Orders," *Associated Press*, 23 June 2005

4 Glassman, James K, and John R Lott, Jr, "The Drug World's Easy Riders," *The Wall Street Journal*, 23 July 2003

5 Hubbard, William K., "Letter to Gregory Gonot," *FDA*, 25 August 2003

6 New Jersey Citizen Action and The Citizen Policy & Education Fund of NJ, "The Drug Company Habit: A Study of Pharmaceutical Industry Campaign Contributions and Policy Influence," 23 September 2003, available online at http://www.njcitizenaction.org/drugcampaignreport.html

7 Davis, Kristin W, "Are Prescriptions Filled in Canada Safe?" *Kiplinger's*, 2004, available online at http://moneycentral.msn.com/content/Insurance/Insureyourhealth/P91657.asp

8 Panos Kanavos, David Gross, and David Taylor, "Parallel Trading in Medicines: Europe's Experience and Its Implications for Commercial Drug Importation in the United States," *AARP*, accessed June 2005, available online at http://www.aarp.org/ppi

9 Glassman, James K, and John R Lott, Jr, "The Drug World's Easy Riders," *The Wall Street Journal*, 23 July 2003

10 H. L. Mencken, *Metalaw*

11 "FDA Test Results of Prescription Drugs from Bogus Canadian website Show All Products Are Fake and Substandard," *FDA News*, accessed 13 July 2004, available online at http://www.fda.gov/fdac/features/2004/404_generic.html

12 Hubbard, "Letter"

13 Horowitz, "Letter"

14 Lueck, Sarah, "FDA Defends Tougher Stance On Drug Imports From Canada," *The Wall Street Journal*, 4 April 2003

15 Horowitz, "Letter"

16 Hubbard, "Letter"

17 "Report: Many Online Pharmacies Posing as Canadian," *iHealthBeat*, 15 June 2005, available online at http://www.ihealth-beat.org/index.cfm?Action=dspItem&itemID=112107

18 Sweet, Lynn, "Illinois Defying Feds, Importing Rx Drugs," *Chicago Sun-Times*, 17 August 2004
19 Davis, "Canada Safe?"
20 Ibid
21 Lannan, Maura Kelly, "Business Slow on State Prescription Drug websites," *Associated Press*, 24 April 2005
22 Hubbard, William K, "Letter to Governor Pawlenty," *FDA*, 24 May 2004, available online at http://www.fda.gov/importeddrugs/pawlenty0524.html
23 Davis, "Canada Safe?"
24 Ibid
25 "Canada Plans to Restrict Internet Drug Orders," *Associated Press*, 23 June 2005, available online at http:/online.wsj.com/article/0,,SB111958271942168611,00.html

Chapter 13: SPECIAL SENIOR REPORT: Medicare Part D Prescription Drug Coverage

1 "Description of the Medicare Prescription Drug Program," *Social Security Administration*, accessed 27 August 2005, available online at http://policy.ssa.gov/poms.nsf/Inx/0603001001
2 "Late Enrollment Penalty Calculation," *MMA Final Regulations Discussion: Sec. 423.286 Rules Regarding Premiums*.
3 Lueck, Sarah, "As Spending Surges, Officials Claim Assets of Estates To Recoup Nursing Costs," *The Wall Street Journal*, 24 June 2005, A1
4 Pear, Robert, "Medicare Change Will Limit Access to Claim Hearing," *New York Times*, 24 April 2005
5 Ibid
6 "Overview of the Medicare Prescription Drug Benefit MMA Title 1 Summary Subpart B—Eligibility, Election and Enrollment," available online at www.cms.hhs.gov/medicarereform/pdbma/TitleIIndex.pdf

ABOUT THE AUTHOR

STEPHEN S. S. HYDE is the founder and CEO of Hyde Rx Services Corp., which provides low-cost prescription drug benefits to companies all over the United States. In the 1970s he founded Peak Health Care, one of the nation's earliest and most successful HMOs, and many of his innovations are still being used today.

INDEX

Exelon, 254–55
eye medications, 254–55

F

Famvir, 145, 241
FDA (Food and Drug
Administration):
and Canadian drugs, 171,
176–77, 178
Electronic Orange Book,
92, 219, 258
enforcement priorities of,
177, 180
generic approvals by, 92,
93–95, 124
on herbals and
supplements, 77–78
OTC approval by, 68–69
Federal Poverty Level
(FPL), 129, 132, 195
Femhrt, 237
Femstat, 252
Flagyl, 239
Flexeril, 225
flexible spending accounts
(FSAs), 43
Flomax, 227
Flonase, 223
Flovent, 91, 226, 259
Floxin Otic, 255
Flumadine, 241
Fluoroplex, 229
fluoxetine (Prozac), 24,
101–2, 106, 232, 261
Foradil, 226
formularies, 22–23, 38–39,
54–57
Fosamax, 259
foster care assistance, 130
free drug programs,
131–36

free-market economy, 26,
168–69
free samples, 10, 19, 62,
96, 121–26, 145–46, 163
FTC (Federal Trade
Commission), 78
Fulvicin, 240
fungal infection medicines,
240
Fungoid Crème, 240, 251

G

Gabitril, 248
generic drugs, 4, 23–25,
89–101
brands compared to,
93–95; *see also* brand
name drugs
copayments for, 36, 54,
159
FDA approvals of, 92,
93–95, 124
lower cost brands, 105–8,
125
me-too drugs, 101–2
missing out on, 96–101
monopolies of, 99–100
narrow therapeutic index
drugs, 94–95
no ads for, 24, 99
no free samples of, 20,
124
prices of, 100, 102–3
question for doctor,
59–60
step therapy, 108
and therapeutically similar
drugs, 103–5
Genora, 231
GI drugs, 234–35
ginger, 256